THE FREE MARKET IN MEDICAL CARE

CENTRAL PLANNING
AND CONTROL
VS. FREE MARKET
MECHANISMS IN
MEDICINE

LEO RAY INGLE, M.D

Copyright © 2015 by Leo Ray Ingle, M.D.

Library of Congress Control Number: 2015905084
ISBN: Hardcover 978-1-5035-5882-3
Softcover 978-1-5035-5883-0
eBook 978-1-5035-5884-7

All rights reserved. No part of this book may be reproduced or transmitted in any form or by any means, electronic or mechanical, including photocopying, recording, or by any information storage and retrieval system, without permission in writing from the copyright owner.

Any people depicted in stock imagery provided by Thinkstock are models, and such images are being used for illustrative purposes only. Certain stock imagery © Thinkstock.

Print information available on the last page.

Rev. date: 04/08/2015

To order additional copies of this book, contact:
Xlibris
1-888-795-4274
www.Xlibris.com
Orders@Xlibris.com
705430

Contents

PART I
INTRODUCTION

Section 1	Overview	3
Section 2	Traditional Free Market	6
Section 3	The Western Model: Greek Medicine	9
Section 4	The Western Model: Medieval Medicine	10

Part II
SCIENTIFIC AND TECHNOLOGICAL ADVANCES IN MEDICINE

Section 5	Scientific and Technological Advances in Medical Care	14
Section 6	Developing and Deploying Technology	26
Section 7	Technology for People as Well as for Profit	27

PART III

Section 8	Best Medical Practice	31

PART IV

Section 9	Research	37

PART V
DELIVERY OF MEDICAL CARE—CENTRAL PLANNING

Section 10	Changes in the Delivery of Medical Care	47
Section 11	Central Planning in Provision of Medical Care	53
Section 12	Central Regulation of Medical Care	57

PART VI
DELIVERY OF MEDICAL CARE-FREE MARKET MECHANISMS

Section 13	The Free Market 69
Section 14	Challenges to Free Market Mechanisms: Challenging Central Planning, Governmental or Corporate 72
Section 15	Challenges to Free Market Mechanisms: Demographic Changes Resulting in Escalating Costs 75
Section 16	Challenges to Free Market Mechanisms: Technology Resulting in Escalating Costs 77

PART VII
POSSIBLE SOLUTIONS

Section 17	Consumer Driven Health Care 82
Section 18	Delivery Of Medical Care-Physician's Role 85
Section 19	Choice for Physicians: Aesculapius or Mercury 88
Section 20	Patients and Doctors 90
Section 21	Physician Negotiation with Payers 92

PART VIII
DISTRIBUTED MEDICAL EDUCATION

Section 22	Distributed Medical Education 97

PART IX
ALTERNATIVE TREATMENTS

Section 23	Alternative Treatments 103

PART X
COST CONTAINMENT

Section 24	Cost Containment 111

PART XI

Section 25	Conclusions 117

PART I

INTRODUCTION

SECTION 1

Overview

It's time to *take back our health care,* restoring the traditional free market in medical care. As with any revolution, the revolution in medicine that would constitute taking back our health care would be meaningless if there were no replacement planned and ready. This book, taken in its entirety, describes a replacement system relying on an authentic free market.

The term *doublespeak* has its origin in George Orwell's book, *Nineteen Eighty-Four.* Although the term doublespeak is not used in the book, it is a close relative of one of the book's central concepts, "doublethink." Orwell highlights examples: peace is war; freedom is slavery and; love is hate. In medicine, examples are the capture of phrases, which are then redefined to mean exactly what "the system" wants them to mean. For example, "Best Medical Practice" is redefined to mean what the government, corporations, and academicians want it to mean—a static, measurable, "expert-generated," government-and-insurer-approved entity, instead of the fluid concept which is traditionally part of the medical lexicon. The Red Queen in *Alice in Wonderland* could be expected to say, "Words mean what I say they mean!" But that reality-altering power, when challenged, will fail. Section 8 describes this pirating of "Best Medical Practice." Similarly, "Free Market" is no longer the concept described by Adam Smith in *Wealth of Nations,* but a never ending war of all-against-all, where "the advantage" is not the benign comparative advantage of Smith, but gleanings of greed, snatched by victors in the struggle.

Central Planning and Control vs. Free Market Mechanisms in Medicine, Leo Ingle, M.D., October 10, 2009

The House of Medicine is built on the ever-shifting sands of "Best Medical Practice" and a specific type of research first described in 1948, the Randomized Controlled Trial. It will be seen that "Best Medical Practice," in the governmental, corporate, and academic meaning, changes with too great a rapidity to be of much utility. "Best Medical Practice," as determined by the free market (and not by government, by corporations, or by academicians), is sufficiently fluid to keep up with changing science and technology.

As discussed in Section 9, the results of Randomized Controlled Trials (RCTs) cannot replace observational studies, observation, or anecdote. The judgment of clinicians is a far better guide. Medical practice must rely on a variety of inputs.

There are several themes running through this book. The most prominent theme is the restoration of a genuine free market in medical care—not the "market" touted by corporations, but a market more akin to the traditional free market and Greek and medieval medical care. Even free markets operate under constraints, the fewer the better—these have traditionally included science and humanitarian and ethical concerns.

The context today includes the amazing scientific and technological advances in medicine, as well as the systems for their development and deployment. Medicine, in utilizing technological advances, needs to consider people as well as profit. Technology is treated in Section 5, Section 6, and Section 7.

Changes in the delivery of medical care have resulted in increasingly centralized control and regulation of medical care. These changes are considered in Section 10, Section 11, and Section 12. As we have seen, changes in the delivery of medical care have provided challenges to the free market, described in Section 13, and to free market mechanisms, described in Section 14, Section 15, and Section 16.

Changes in the delivery of medical care have resulted in challenges to the independence of doctors (Section 18). Doctors are presented with a choice of serving people or seeking profit (Section 19). The dyad of the physician and the patient, exercising free choice in the universe of options, represents the best chance for restoring the free market in medical care existing before the 1600's (Section 20).

Physicians and physician groups must be free to negotiate payment from government and corporate payers (Section 21).

Cost containment will be effective and real only in the context of this restored free market in medical care (Section 24).

Section 2

Traditional Free Market

Traditional medicine provided services in a market environment

Traditionally, medicine had been a profession or guild, providing services in a market environment. Provision of services was primarily on the basis of free market principles. Price generally varied depending on the elements of supply and demand. Medical care began with a patient's verbal history and an examination of the body part. The individual physician then did everything possible to provide rapid relief.

The Hippocratic Oath, a form of which is still frequently taken by graduating physicians, is believed to have been written by Hippocrates, the Father of Western Medicine, in Greece, in the 5th century BC. The traditional form included the following language:

> I swear by Apollo the physician and Aesculapius the surgeon, likewise Hygeia and Panacea, and all the gods and goddesses to witness that I will observe and keep this underwritten oath, to the utmost of my power and judgment.
>
> With regard to healing the sick, I will devise and order for them the best diet, according to my judgment and means; and I will take care that they suffer no hurt or

damage. I will comport myself and use my knowledge in a godly manner.

Whatever house I may enter; my visit shall be for the convenience and advantage of the patient. Whatever in the course of my practice, I may see or hear (even when not invited), whatever I may happen to obtain knowledge of, if it be not proper to repeat it, I will keep sacred and secret within my own breast.

If I faithfully observe this oath, may I thrive and prosper in my fortune and profession, and live in estimation of posterity; or on breach thereof may the reverse be my fate!"[1]

This relic of remote antiquity has for many years slipped from the common view of the profession. We cannot imagine that affording it a place here can give offense elsewhere.

Legitimate non-market constraints on medical care have included science, humanitarian concerns, and medical ethics

Non-market constraints and limits on provision of medical services have always existed. Perhaps the single greatest constraint, even before the Enlightenment, was the appearance and actuality of the utility of that care. Utility, including both efficacy and safety, has been most frequently defined in terms of either a supernatural or a scientific system. With the Enlightenment and the increasing replacement of the supernatural system by the scientific system, came a more vigorous application of scientific method and reason to the analysis of the efficacy and safety of medical interventions.

Non-market constraints have, in the past, included humanitarian concerns. An example of that sort of concern would include the following incident from the medical treatment of the insane: In 1795, at the Salpêtrière (Bicêtre) Asylum in Paris, Philippe Pinel released what were then called "lunatics" from their chains. In the lobby of the Paris Academy of Medicine, a large painting, eighteen by eight foot, depicts

---

[1] "The Hippocratic Oath," The London Medical Repository 23, no. 135 (1825): 258.

the event. Too little is written about the entire professional career of this founder of French psychiatry, but perhaps too much about this one act. Philippe Pinel was motivated by humanitarian concerns, not scientific concerns.

Non-market constraints have, in the past, included medical ethics.

With increasing vertical organization, regulation, and control in the modern system, it is difficult to find surviving examples of the traditional free market. One example that comes to mind is the farmer's markets held regularly in many communities. Farmers bring local produce to the market which is attended by customers who appreciate the quality and price of the goods. Farmers have booths to display and sell. The principal regulation, sporadically enforced if at all, is that the producer must be the seller. The sales tax is collected and remitted by the seller. Customers have a choice of vendor, and, over time, the elements of quality and price drive out the noncompetitive vendors. There is certainly no "predetermined price" for, say, a cabbage or a pear. Vegetables vary in quality and size.

Compare that to the "modern" health care system, where choice of provider is limited, and where payment is made most frequently to an insurer whose "administrative costs" are, on average, about 30 percent. Costs are further driven up by the requirement that the doctor complete time-consuming "paperwork" to justify and collect his or her fee. The fee is not set in a competitive way, but is determined in advance based upon "diagnosis." Farmer's markets have more inherent wisdom than this—a cabbage is not just any old cabbage; a pear is not just any old pear.

SECTION 3

The Western Model: Greek Medicine

The Western "Medical Model" is derived from the model developed by the Greeks. The Greeks created rational medicine, though the work of succeeding "schools" was not often entirely scientific in the modern sense of the term. In *Aspects of Greek Medicine*,[2] E.D. Phillips traces the development of professional medicine from its earliest beginnings through the Hippocratic corpus, thence to the Alexandrian school, and finally, to Galen. The philosophic background to this progression is discussed, as philosophic attitudes influenced medicine then as now. Had the free market aspects of Greek medicine survived, we would not have the present irrational variance in charges and costs. Throughout this period, medical care was individualized to the patient, with examination not limited to the "complaint." Although treatment range was limited and awaited scientific advancement, as well as development and deployment of technology, the methods of delivery of care were sound.

---

[2] E.D. Phillips, *Aspects of Greek Medicine* (New York: St. Martin's Press, 1973).

Section 4

The Western Model: Medieval Medicine

The Western "Medical Model" owes much to the medieval practice of medicine. Modern medicine did not emerge until the 1600's. William Harvey (1578–1657) made great progress in understanding the anatomy and physiology of the human body, especially of the circulatory system, largely by dissecting cadavers. Anton van Leeuwenhoek (1632–1723) developed microscopes, greatly enlarging the observable world.

A millennium ago, most of the population lived in small villages where there was always a healer who was the antecedent of the family practitioner or country doctor. The healer or "family practitioner" often knew his patients from infancy, since he had delivered them. He made house calls. He knew the physical and familial context of every illness.

During the entire period before modern medicine, the prominence of free market mechanisms and individualized care by practitioners characterized medical care.

Part II

SCIENTIFIC AND TECHNOLOGICAL ADVANCES IN MEDICINE

In Part II, Section 5, we will explore scientific and technological advances in medical care. We will describe the history of these advances in the field of medical care. We will also introduce the concept and term "technocapitalism." We will describe multiple effects of these scientific and technological advances in changing the role of physicians and in increasing costs of care. Areas of technology, to include medical devices, vaccines, and drugs will be discussed. The effect on medical care of computers and electronic medical records will likewise be discussed.

In Part II, Section 6, we will discuss the development and deployment of technological advances.

In Part II, Section 7, we introduce the dichotomy of patients versus profits.

SECTION 5

Scientific and Technological Advances in Medical Care

We are in the middle of a Technological Revolution which rivals the Industrial Revolution in significance. It is an overwhelming task to consider the character and effect of technological advances even in a limited area such as health care. Technological advances have dramatically changed the role of the primary care physician and have changed the delivery of health care in every specialty, medical or surgical.

Moreover, the relationship between technology and economics in the United States has given rise to an entirely new phenomenon and a new term, that is, technocapitalism. Luis Suarez-Villa, a professor in the School of Social Ecology at the University of California in Irvine, has been highly critical of technocapitalism in his book by that title:

> Technocapitalism is defined in this book as a new form of capitalism that is heavily grounded on corporate power and its exploitation of technological creativity. Creativity, an intangible human quality, is the most precious resource of this new incarnation of capitalism. Corporate power and profit inevitably depend on the commodification of creativity through research regimes that must generate new inventions and innovations.

> These regimes and the corporate apparatus in which they are embedded are to technocapitalism what the factory system and its production regimes were to industrial capitalism.[3]

Even for those of us committed to a major role for corporations and capital in a free market economy, many of Luis Suarez-Villa's criticisms ring true.

The Technological Revolution has caused, in conjunction with our corporate structures, massive change in the delivery of health care. Just as in the Industrial Revolution, unfortunate effects and abuses had to be reined in by governmental action, so too, in the Technological Revolution, unfortunate effects and abuses will need to be reined in.

Technological advances in medicine

Prior to 1900, limitations in both efficacy and safety of medical science prevented the development of hospitals as we know them. Hospices existed principally for the critically ill poor. Asylums existed for the insane.

Prior to 1900, limitations in both efficacy and safety of medical procedures and drugs held down both their price and their use.

Medical science emerged in the 15th and 16th centuries. During the early 17th century, the English doctor, William Harvey (1578–1657), made important advances in understanding the workings of the human body. After studying medicine with the Italian surgeon, Fabricius (1537–1619; also known as Fabrici), Harvey conducted experiments to determine the flow of blood by dissecting (cutting apart piece by piece to study) cadavers (dead bodies used for scientific study). Harvey learned that the heart pumps blood through the arteries to all parts of the body and that the blood returns through the veins to the heart. In 1628, he published his findings in *An Anatomical Study on the Motion of the Heart and the Blood in Animals*. Building on this and later works, the twin, basic sciences of anatomy and physiology emerged as the core of our medical curriculum.

---

[3] Luis Suarez-Villa, *Technocapitalism: A Critical Perspective on Technological Innovation and Corporatism* (Philadelphia: Temple University Press, 2009), 3.

Another pivotal development in medicine came when Anton van Leeuwenhoek (1632–1723), a Dutch naturalist, developed microscopes so he could study objects invisible to the naked eye, including bacteria. This discovery was a major milestone in medical knowledge, spurring major advances in the diagnosis and treatment of infectious diseases.

Every subsequent century brought advances in medical science and application of that science to the diagnosis and treatment of patients. During the 20th century, the rate of change climbed more steeply. Medicine at the beginning of the 21st century looked nothing like medicine at the beginning of the 20th century.

Technological advances in medicine and surgery allowed the previously rare concept of "cure" to emerge as a goal.

Infectious diseases that, before the 20th century, disabled and killed millions can now be prevented by supplying clean water, by improving sanitation, and by vaccination. Those resisting prevention can be treated with antibiotics. Technological advances in public health, immunization, and antibiotics prevent untold suffering and pain. The average expected life span in the United States increased from 47.3 years in 1900 to 77.0 years in 2000.[4] Pre-Columbian Indians are thought to have had expected life spans of 25 to 30 years.[5]

Vaccine-preventable diseases include anthrax, diphtheria, hepatitis A and B, influenza, measles, meningococcal meningitis, mumps, pertussis (whooping cough), pneumococcal pneumonia, polio, rabies, rubella, shingles, smallpox, tetanus, typhoid, tuberculosis, varicella (chickenpox), and yellow fever.[6]

The discovery of sulfonamide antibiotics by Gerhard Domagk (who received the Nobel Prize for Medicine in 1939) and the discovery of

---

[4] "National Vital Statistics Report," Volume 56, No. 9 (December 28, 2007). Figures for 1900 (47.3) through 1929 (59.1) are from death registration states only. Life expectancy in the United States increased from 59.7 years in 1930, to 62.9 years in 1940, to 68.2 years in 1950, to 69.7 years in 1960, to 70.8 years in 1970, to 73.7 years in 1980, to 75.4 years in 1990, and to 77.0 years in 2000.

[5] Pre-European Exploration, Pre-History through 1540.

[6] Center for Disease Control, June 12, 2007.

penicillin antibiotics by Alexander Fleming (who shared the Nobel Prize for Medicine in 1945 with Howard Florey and Ernst Chain who purified penicillin for clinical use) began a series of advances in the treatment of infectious disease.[7]

Antibiotics are divided into those that are time-dependent, like the beta-lactams and vancomycin and those that are concentration-dependent, including the aminoglycosides, fluoroquinolones, and metronidazole. Many more are time-dependent but concentration-enhanced, such as the macrolides, clindamycin, tetracycline, minocyclines, and clindamycin. Antibiotics work through a variety of mechanisms, including blockage of cell wall synthesis, cell membrane disruption, interference with DNA replication and messenger RNA synthesis, interference with folic acid synthesis, and interference with protein synthesis. The beta-lactams include the penicillins, such as amoxicillin and ampicillin, and the cephalosporins, such as Keflin and Keflex. There are about 30 million reported instances of penicillin allergy, but only about 1.5 million instances of actual allergy.

Public health measures are credited with much of the recent increase in life expectancy. During the 20th century, the average lifespan in the United States increased by more than 30 years, of which 25 years can be attributed to advances in public health.

---

[7] Synthetic antibiotic chemotherapy as a science and the story of antibiotic development began in Germany with Paul Ehrlich, a German medical scientist in the late 1880s. Dr. Ehrlich noted that certain dyes would bind to and color human, animal, or bacterial cells, while others did not. He then extended the idea that it might be possible to make certain dyes or chemicals that would act as a magic bullet or selective drug that would bind to and kill bacteria while not harming the human host. After much experimentation, screening hundreds of dyes against various organisms, he discovered a medicinally useful drug, the man-made antibiotic, Salvarsan. However, the adverse side effect profile of salvarsan, coupled with the later discovery of the antibiotic penicillin, superseded its use as an antibiotic. The work of Ehrlich, which marked the birth of the antibiotic revolution, was followed by the discovery of prontosil by Domagk in 1932.

Technology gnawed away at the physician's role in the healing process

Technological advances, however, came at a price. Physicians, already handmaidens to the entrepreneurial aspects of their practices, became, in addition, handmaidens to technology, machines, devices, and drugs. Technology gnawed away at the physician's role as a healer. The physical presence of doctors became less and less important.

The physician's "black bag" fell into disfavor, to be replaced by a prescription pad. Perhaps the most ubiquitous technological change was that "patent medicines" ceased to be an epithet describing elixirs, capsules, or pills sold from the back of "medicine wagons" by unscrupulous vendors. Those elixirs, containing "medicines" like paregoric[8] and alcohol, otherwise had a placebo effect and little additional effect, good or bad. Giant pharmaceutical companies now promoted, with immense profit, proprietary drugs that remain under patent for many years. "Detailers" fan out from those pharmaceutical companies to hospitals and clinics all over the country, promoting recent "advances in medicine," by which they mean new patent drugs.

I began my practice of medicine in Bessemer, Alabama, in 1969, with two other doctors. Our basic charge for an office visit was seven dollars at that place and time. The reputation of penicillin (in the form of injectable AP-Bicillin or oral V-Cillin K) was such that most patients, whether suffering from a bacterial infection or not, wanted the shot. The doctor down the street, who charged only five dollars, would, without examination, simply provide the shot (of penicillin). I became so exasperated with this medically indefensible demand for "a shot" that, when a drug salesman came through offering an injectable mix of eucalyptus oil and oil of cajeput, both aromatic oils producing a scent-laden breath when injected, I bought a supply. Ultimately, I neither injected the eucalyptus oil and oil of cajeput mix, nor an alternative injection—a pretty red vitamin B12 shot.

---

[8] Paregoric is a mixture of powdered opium, anise oil, benzoic acid, camphor, and glycerin in diluted alcohol, used as an antiperistaltic, especially in the treatment of diarrhea, or as an analgesic for pain.

Role of capital in the development of new technology in medical care

In a competitive free market system, there is a continual effort on the part of competitors to improve the technical forces of production in order to maximize profits by lowering costs. In the medical industry, unlike industries where standardized commodities are more ubiquitous, technological progress tends to increase costs, rather than to lower costs.

With the emergence of a medical industry, the role of corporations in the delivery of health care increased dramatically, both in the payment for health care by insurance companies and in the delivery of health care. At the beginning of my medical practice, the corporate practice of medicine was anathema, but constraints on corporate practice, thinly disguised by the licensure of physician employees, have been eroding for three decades.

Corporations, though interpreted as having characteristics of persons beginning with the United States Supreme Court's announcement in 1886,[9] and extended over the years, differ from physicians in

---

[9] Below is the 1886 Supreme Court decision granting corporations the same rights as living persons under the Fourteenth Amendment to the Constitution. Quoting from David Korten's *The Post-Corporate World, Life After Capitalism* (pp.185-6):
In 1886, . . . in the case of *Santa Clara County v. Southern Pacific Railroad Company*, the U.S. Supreme Court decided that a private corporation is a person and entitled to the legal rights and protections the Constitutions affords to any person. The doctrine of corporate personhood, which subsequently became a cornerstone of corporate law, was introduced into this 1886 decision without argument. According to the official case record, Supreme Court Justice Morrison Remick Waite simply pronounced before the beginning of argument in the case of *Santa Clara County v. Southern Pacific Railroad Company* that: "The court does not wish to hear argument on the question whether the provision in the Fourteenth Amendment to the Constitution, which forbids a State to deny to any person within its jurisdiction the equal protection of the laws, applies to these corporations. We are all of opinion that it does."
The court reporter duly entered into the summary record of the Court's findings that:

significant respects. The motivation of corporations is, as an agent of the stockholders, to maximize profit, and only secondarily and to the extent it increases corporate profits, to provide efficacious and safe medical care. Individual corporate representatives and agents may have consciences, but the corporation, as such, does not. Physicians, on the other hand, are members of a profession, licensed to provide efficacious and safe medical care. In my experience, my fellow physicians, despite erosion of their role, still, generally, following a professional code of medical ethics, place patient care first, ahead of making money.

Corporations have, across the United States, shifted from an industrial model to a technology model in the evolving marketplace. The new model has been called technocapitalism. The medical industry needs to be considered in the context of that emerging technological model.

University, government, and corporate research all produced patentable new technology. These technologies, especially with their patents, provide an entrepreneurial opportunity for investors, corporate and individual. Investors can count on a high rate of return. Due to the patent system, companies do not have to be concerned about competition and competitive pricing.

Dr. Thomas Kuhn published a book, *The Structure of Scientific Revolutions,* in 1962, stating that the development of scientific research was grounded in social structures. Dr. Kuhn believed that for each scientific discipline, a paradigm exists that involves both the way the discipline is envisioned and the way change occurs. In medicine, as in physics, chemistry, and biology dominant explanations hold sway. Research is done from within the established paradigm. Professional publication depends on peer review and is limited almost always to papers adhering to established research protocols and ideas.

" The defendant Corporations are persons within the intent of the clause in section 1 of the Fourteen Amendment to the Constitution of the United States, which forbids a State to deny to any person within its jurisdiction the equal protection of the laws."

Thus it was that a two-sentence assertion by a single judge elevated corporations to the status of persons under the law, prepared the way for the rise of global corporate rule, and thereby changed the course of history. This file is mirrored from: http://laws.findlaw.com/us/118/394.html.

The dominant paradigm over time is challenged by newer paradigms, newer processes, and newer ideas. In medicine, these challenges almost always accompany the development of a new technology.

Medical technology, as distinct from medical science, has advanced in tandem with the development of diagnostic technology, medical devices, and drugs.

Development of diagnostic technology has been rapid, especially in the area of medical imaging, to include MRIs and CTs.

New treatment technologies exist in surgery and anesthesia, including expansion of laparoscopic surgery and development of transplantation and bypass systems. Interventional cardiology developed with advances in arteriography, including coronary arteriography, and with ever more frequent placement of stents. The field of medical devices expanded to include such diverse items as coronary pacemakers and metal or metal-carbon replacements for joints, to include the hip and knee. Medical devices can be categorized according to risk:

High risk devices are those whose failure or misuse is reasonable likely to seriously injure patients or staff, examples include:

- Anesthesia ventilators
- Anesthesia units
- Apnea monitors
- Argon enhanced coagulation units
- Aspirators
- Autotransfusion units
- Invasive blood pressure units
- Fetal monitors
- Electrosurgical units
- Incubators
- Infusion pump
- Pulse oximeters
- External pacemaker
- Heart-lung machine

Medium risk devices are those whose misuse, failure, or absence (e.g., out of service) with no replacement available would have a significant impact on patient care, but would not be likely to cause direct serious injury. Examples include:

- ECG
- EEG
- Treadmills
- Ultrasound sensors
- Phototherapy units
- Endoscopes
- Surgical drill and saws
- Laparoscopic insufflators
- Phonocardiographs
- Radiant warmers (adult)
- Zoophagous agents (e.g., medicinal leeches; medicinal maggots)
- Lytic bacteriophages

Low risk devices are those whose failure or misuse is unlikely to result in serious consequences. Examples include:

- Electronic thermometer
- Breast pumps
- Surgical microscope
- Ultrasonic nebulizers
- Sphygmomanometers
- Surgical table
- Surgical lights
- Temperature monitor
- Aspirators
- X-rays diagnostic equipment

A major advance in medicine, as distinct from surgery, has been in the area of drugs, patentable and profitable.

Another major advance has been the development of vaccines, available for all the vaccine-preventable diseases. These include:

- Anthrax
- Cervical cancer
- Diptheria
- Hepatitis A
- Hepatitis B

- Haemophilus influenzae, Type B
- Human papillomavirus
- Influenza
- Japanese encephalitis
- Lyme disease
- Measles
- Meningococcal meningitis
- Mumps
- Pertussis
- Pneumococcal pneumonia
- Polio
- Rabies
- Rubella
- Shingles smallpox
- Tetanus
- Typhoid
- Tuberculosis
- Varicella
- Yellow fever

Computers are in widespread use in surveillance and control of medical care. The electronic medical record (EMR) or electronic health record (EHR) provide templates for recording details of patient diagnosis and treatment in digital format. The electronic record can, theoretically, be shared across a number of health care settings.

While one study reported an overall efficiency saving of 6 percent by adoption of EMRs, a 2014 survey of an American College of Physicians member sample found that physicians spent forty-eight minutes more a day on EMRs. Ninety percent reported that at least one data management function was slower after EMRs were adopted and 64 percent reported that note writing took longer. Thirty-four percent reported it took longer to find and review medical data and 32 percent reported that it was slower to read other clinicians notes.[10]

According to the Privacy Rights Clearinghouse's Chronology of Data Security Breaches involving medical information, medical and health care providers have experienced 767 security breaches resulting in the

---

[10] Clement McDonald, et al., "Use of Internist's Free Time by Ambulatory Care Electronic Medical Records Systems," *JAMA Internal Medicine* 174, no. 11 (2014): 1860–1863.

compromised confidential health information of 23,625,933 patients during the period 2006 to 2012.

Electronic medical records can be easily searched and compiled. Paper medical charts are not. In 1990, I undertook to survey a random sample of our clinic charts—a sample size of 100. Despite my considerable skills at deriving information from medical charts and in scanning, I required almost an hour per chart to retrieve and enter the desired data.

The existence of electronic medical records allows easy surveillance of large amounts of data, being eminently searchable and compilable. They are an essential element in the centralized regulation and control of medicine. Guidelines and algorithms cease to be suggestions and become enforceable. Individual physicians can be measured for compliance with mandates for extent and type of care.

Technological advances included important changes in testing. Some blood tests are pathognomonic of a particular disease, as, for example, the hemoglobin A1c and the blood sugars, fasting and postprandial, for diabetes. When, however, certain blood tests were mindlessly linked to a diagnosis and a treatment, errors arise. For example, the thyroid stimulating hormone (TSH) is still used to "determine" the presence or absence of hyperthyroidism and hypothyroidism. Clinical symptoms and signs are often not considered. The recipe is: If the TSH is high, the circulating effective thyroid hormone is low, and if the TSH is low, the circulating effective thyroid hormone is high. This bypasses the complex relationship between T3 and T4, and the amount of protein binding. Doctors have come to rely on testing, to the exclusion of important medical history and physical findings.

Imaging studies are similarly flawed. Over two decades ago, I saw three neurosurgeons who recommended surgery for my cervical disks. They asserted that my MRI was absolute proof of my need for surgery. I called the radiologist who had read my MRI, asking for an appointment. He questioned why I would want to see him, but, when I reminded him that I was his patient and he was my doctor, he agreed. He questioned the payment, and I told him I would pay his fee by check or cash. At first, sitting in his office, he was reluctant to talk, until I pledged not to disclose what he said to anyone, especially to the neurosurgeons he depended on for referrals. He placed my MRI on the screen and pointed out the apparent narrowing or the intervertebral disk space and blockage of the foramen. I asked him, "What does this mean?" He went back to his records room, and brought another MRI, which appears far more "damaged" than mine. He pointed out that it was his MRI, and that he had never had symptoms. There is no certain relationship between MRI findings and the clinical picture or the need for surgery. I have been symptom-free for years though. I never got surgery.

Section 6

Developing and Deploying Technology

Government financing, as distinct from corporate financing, of research has the luxury of focusing on the long-range acquisition of knowledge rather than the search for short-range profit.

Research can be divided into studies directed to the long-term, usually government-funded, and studies directed to the short-term. Both categories lead to the development of new advances, be they medical devices or drugs. Deployment of these new technologies is far more dependent on their profitability than their efficacy and safety. Profitability determines the intensity of marketing efforts on the part of makers of drugs and devices. Successive maps showing deployment are similar, which spread from early adoption centers to wider areas, taking over a decade to reach most of the country. Thus, "Best Medical Practice" will depend on geography—with late adopters lagging sometimes over twenty years. The difference between early adopters and late adopters depends a lot on physician age. Older physicians are slow to change.

Peter Orszag, then director of the White House Office of Management and Budget, wrote in a column in the October 10, 2010 issue of the New York Times, that, "One estimate suggests that it takes seventeen years to incorporate new research findings into widespread practice."

Section 7

Technology for People as Well as for Profit

Clearly, from the preceding discussion, there is a divergence in considering technology as a way of improving health care and as a way to make profits.

Corporations are, by and large, driven by profit. People want improved health care. Consumers of medical care rely on traditional "healing methods" taught by parents or part of the general knowledge pool. Often, these healing methods have no scientific basis. Reliance on the Internet, though more current, has little to offer the patient. People need an "ombudsperson" to assist them in steering between the Scylla of entrepreneurial gain and the Charybdis of technology, inadequately vetted. That ombudsperson can be, and often is, the physician. The ombudsperson is helpful to the degree he or she is (1) independent of financial entanglements; (2) aware, through continuing education or the current state of medical science; (3) concerned for the welfare of the patient; and, finally, (4) ethical.

PART III

Section 8

Best Medical Practice

"Best Medical Practice" is not what the ordinary person would intuit, the best treatment for an individual in a particular context. Instead, it is the linking of a standardized *treatment* with a *diagnosis*. Thus, the concept of diagnosis is reified, considered to be a "thing itself" rather than a general description of a variable constellation of symptoms and signs. This reified ("thingified," if you will) diagnosis is linked to an unvarying treatment. The "Best Medical Practice" might apply to anywhere from a bare majority of sufferers to a much higher percentage.

In addition, the "Best Medical Practice" changes with time. Contradictory evidence reverses "best practices" so frequently that within one year, 15 percent must be changed, within two years, 23 percent are reversed, and at 5.5 years, half are incorrect.[11]

Samuel Arbesman has generalized this finding in *The Half-Life of Facts: Why Everything We Know Has an Expiration Date*.[12] He divides facts along a spectrum. At one end are ephemeral facts, like the current time, and at the other are relatively constant facts, like the number of fingers on a human hand. The vast middle contains "mesofacts," which change at

---

[11] Kaveh G. Shojana, et al., "How Quickly Do Systemic Reviews Go Out of Date: A Survival Analysis," *Annals of Internal Medicine* (August 21, 2007).

[12] Samuel Arbesman, *The Half Life of Facts: Why Everything We Know Has an Expiration Date* (New York: Current [a member of Penguin Group USA], 2012).

a middle timescale. This results in a decay of knowledge, occurring at more or less a predictable rate. For example, the truth of knowledge in the areas of hepatitis and cirrhosis declined 50 percent in around forty-five years. It takes forty-five years for half the knowledge in these fields to be overturned.[13]

After the introduction of a drug or a medical device, subsequent findings in widespread practice modify their role in medical practice. There are many examples in the area of pharmacology. One such is Zithromax (azithromycin), a drug prescribed for, among other infections, bronchitis, which was found to cause cardiac deaths in a small percentage of patients. Patients with heart disease should avoid Zithromax. Lap-Bands, surgical mesh, and metal hips have all been shown to have safety problems not initially reported.

The concept of "Best Medical Practice" involves the use of "algorithms" or guidelines for practice, which are then statistically compared. The mathematics and statistics utilized, though often internally consistent, can have little or no relationship to reality.

The evidence behind "Evidence-Based Medicine" is both limited and faulty.

Philosophers have, since the time of Immanuel Kant, emphasized that we are not born into a common, structured world apparent to us all, but that we each perceive the world in our unique way.

Postmodern philosophers have taken that particular ball and run with it.

But positivism and science soldier on.

Science is described as dealing with ever more accurate hypotheses about the existing world, allowing ever more accurate predictions of future events. This suggests an "end point" that exists, though never reached.

The mathematical model of calculus does allow for manipulation of end points that are not specifiable or known, but can be symbolized. The

---

[13] Poynard, et al., "Truth Survival in Clinical Research: An Evidence Based Requiem?" *Annals of Internal Medicine* 136, no. 12 (2002): 888–895.

mathematician is confident enough in the existence of those end points that they are used in equations describing scientific reality.

Analogously, according to this argument, although none of us can be confident that our perceived world is the real world, we stand on the shoulders of intellectual giants, present and past, who approximated that "real world." With enough such approximations, can we, finally, be able to develop a usable understanding of the real world?

This thinking has a lot in common with the concepts behind "fuzzy logic." In fuzzy logic, every fact comes with a percentage—estimating the likelihood that the fact represents reality.

How closely does the mental, including mathematics and statistics, correspond to the real?

At best, there is an asymptotic approach of those mental metaphors and images tending toward, but never reaching, "the real."

Thus, the argument goes, the aggregate of scientific knowledge is progressing to an ever better understanding of the world around us. As part of this process, we asymptotically approach the truth.[14] Even this asymptotic level of certainty is denied us, however.

In 1736, Thomas Bayes published a mathematics paper that immortalized him in the field of statistics—and medical tests.[15] He mathematically proved his theory of conditional probability—to understand something's meaning, we have to understand its context. For example, medical tests are only correct in the context of who gets tested.[16]

Further, Werner Heisenberg developed his Uncertainty Principle in the years before 1926. According to that principle, knowledge gained in physical sciences is limited in ways we have yet to grasp.[17]

---

[14] Arbesman, *The Half Life of Facts*, 36–37.

[15] David H. Newman, MD, *Hippocrates' Shadow: Secrets from the House of Medicine: What Doctors Don't Know, Don't Tell You, and How Truth Can Repair the Patient-Doctor Breach* (New York: Scribner, 2008).

[16] Ibid., 202.

[17] Ibid., 204.

Five years later, Kurt Gödel published his paper, "On Formally Undecidable Propositions of Principia Mathematica and Related Systems."[8]

Neither mathematics nor science are true outside of their domains or context.

Uncertain Inference, by Henry Kyburg and Choh Man Teng, explores uncertainty and uncertain inference in depth. All interesting inference is uncertain. It is uncertain in one or both of two ways. Either some of the propositions on which the conclusion is based are uncertain, in which case that uncertainty contaminates the conclusion, or (more often) both some of the premises and the principle of inference lead to uncertainty.[19]

---

[18] Ibid., 205.

[19] Henry Kyburg and Choh Man Teng, *Uncertain Inference* (United Kingdom: Cambridge University Press, 2001), 286.

PART IV

Section 9

Research

In our enthusiasm about the benefits we have derived from the Enlightenment, the scientific method, and science, we endorse research—especially anointing peer-reviewed Randomized Controlled Trials (RCT) as a reflection of "the state of the art." The Randomized Controlled Trial (RCT) is a relative newcomer to science which for centuries depended on observation and measurement. The first published RCT appeared in a 1948 study entitled "Streptomycin treatment of pulmonary tuberculosis." One of the authors of that paper was Austin Hill who is credited as having conceived the modern RCT.

Science and scientific evidence, observation, and measurement have been at the heart of monumental advances in medical and surgical care, beginning and continuing during centuries when observational evidence and simple trials were all there was.

In coming to conclusions in science, we use all types of evidence. Scientific conclusions are based on a consilience of all sorts of evidence and data, different, even disparate.[20]

The science of medicine in the last two centuries has expanded and enhanced the knowledge of the body and of the pathologic conditions

---

[20] Samuel Scheiner, "Experiments, Observations, and Other Types of Evidence," in *The Nature of Scientific Evidence*, ed. Mark Taper and Subhash Lele (Chicago: University of Chicago Press), 51–69.

which threaten its well-being. The application of that knowledge to treating patients exposed physicians and their patients to a variability inherent in the wide range of conditions. There are intercurrent disorders not taken into account in the research studies. Patient variability, due to environmental and genetic causes, is wide.

The basic principles of the Randomized Controlled Trial (RCT) are widely known. Variables in constructing an RCT include selection of subjects, picking the measurements that will be made throughout the trial and specifying how they will be made, and specifying when the trial will end. Some RCTs have follow-up, many do not.

The RCT has been widely said to be the gold standard. Can it be, in practice, a kind of fool's gold? While the reproducibility of seminal research studies that have been done has been called into question, that reproducibility is touted as a cardinal characteristic of the RCT. Reproducibility is a cardinal element for precision. Even if reproducible and precise, are the findings of RCTs accurate? *Accuracy* is a term meaning the consistency of findings with the real world. Accuracy, unlike precision, cannot be improved by such simple devices as increasing the sample size.

We must never forget that the RCT is a newcomer on the scientific scene, developed in 1948. It has not changed over the last seven decades. We know that science can proceed without it.

For better or worse, the Randomized Controlled Trial or RCT, a specific type of scientific experiment or trial, appears to have eclipsed all other methods. The RCT is used to test the efficacy and safety of various types of intervention within a patient population. Study subjects, before the intervention begins, are randomly assigned to alternative groups, comparing treatment groups with a group not receiving treatment (as in a placebo controlled study).

RCTs can be classified as either explanatory or pragmatic. The explanatory RCT tests efficacy in a structured research setting with highly selected subjects under highly controlled conditions. Such a study cannot inform decisions about practice. Pragmatic RCTs test effectiveness in everyday practice with relatively unselected subjects under flexible conditions and can potentially inform practice.

The randomization process is not without problems. The process of randomization can introduce both accidental and selection biases. Simple randomization in RCTs with fewer than 200 subjects often leads to imbalanced group sizes. There are several popular forms of restricted randomization. In block randomization, allocation ratio and block size are specified for subgroups with random selection within each block. For example, a block size of ten and an allocation ratio of 4:1, would lead to random assignment of eight subjects to one group and two to the other. However, even with large block sizes, this procedure can lead to selection bias. Another form of restricted randomization is adaptive randomization. In adaptive randomization, the probability of assignment to a group changes as the study proceeds.

Allocation concealment is the mechanism for insuring that the treatment to be allocated is not known before subjects are entered into the study. Investigators have frequently introduced both selection bias and confounders by violating protocols to dictate the assignment of their next patient. Methods of ensuring allocation concealment include sequentially numbered opaque sealed envelopes (SNOSE), sequentially numbered containers, pharmacy controlled randomization, and central randomization.

A RCT may be blinded or masked by procedures that prevent study participants and outcome assessors from knowing which intervention was received. Blinding is sometimes inappropriate or impossible. RCTs without blinding are called "unblinded" or "open." Unblinded RCTs tend to be biased toward beneficial effects.

Disadvantages of RCT's include:

1. Applicability to the Real World

RCT's are limited to the "universe" designated by the parameters of the study. Applicability outside of that, frequently narrow universe.

- The location of the RCT varies. An RCT conducted in a "Third World" country like Liberia, may have limited applicability to industrialized countries. Within the industrialized countries, political and social characteristics may limit the applicability, as, for example, a study in Sweden may not fully apply in the United States or Britain.

- Many RCT's are limited to patients who do not have any coexisting medical or psychiatric illnesses. Many choose patients in a limited range of prognosis, as for example, excluding the gravely ill or the minimally ill. Many are limited to adult males, thus excluding women and children. Plavix, after approval based on overall improvement of the test population, was prescribed for years before it came to light that over 30% of the population could not metabolize the drug to the active form. [21]
- The RCT patients often receive a level of observation not typical of "ordinary" patients. That observation and attention often alters the course of the illness, as much as the studied elements. Further, there is a typical assumption that the same dose works for all patients, a "one-dose-fits-all" mentality. [22]
- Often the RCT uses outcome measures that differ from those used in general practice. This can alter the reported results either negatively or positively. Most often it seems, the selected measures permit a better final outcome.
- Often adverse effects are not reported, or not fully reported.

2. Costs

One limitation of the RCT is its cost. Pharmaceutical companies choose to do an RCT, with a total cost averaging over $10 million dollars, only when the expected return during the patent period justifies that outlay. A negative outcome is costly for the company. A positive outcome can result in billions of dollars of income. Company profits and stock price can soar, with a new "blockbuster" drug. Obviously, potential drugs with limited profitability will not be chosen for an RCT. Relatively few are funded through the "orphan" drug program.

3. Time

An RCT takes time to plan and to conduct. Administrative procedures related to approval take time. Practicing doctors do not hear of the

---

[21] The Creative Destruction of Medicine, Eric Topol, M.D., Basic Books, New York, 2012, p. 25.

[22] Ibid, p. 25.

new drug until years after the RCT is begun. Sometimes there is a "rush to market", and a doctor may be faced with a choice of two or more new drugs for the same condition. Lacking information on how they compare, they rely on observation and anecdote.

Two other lines of reasoning question RCTs' contribution to scientific knowledge beyond other types of studies:

If study designs are ranked by their potential for new discoveries, then anecdotal evidence would be at the top of the list, followed by observational studies, followed by RCTs.

RCTs may be unnecessary for treatments that have dramatic and rapid effects relative to the expected stable or progressively worse natural course of the condition treated. One example is combination chemotherapy including cisplatin for metastatic testicular cancer, which increased the cure rate from 5 percent to 60 percent in a 1977 non-randomized study.

In 2005, John Ioannidis published the article "Why Most Published Research Findings Are False" in the journal *PLoS Medicine*,[23] concluding that:

1. The smaller the studies the less likely the research findings are to be true.
2. The smaller the effect the less likely the research findings are to be true.
3. The greater the financial and other interests, the less likely the research findings are to be true.
4. The hotter a scientific field, the less likely the research findings are to be true.

There is a high rate of non-replication of significant research findings. Amgen, an American drug company, tried to replicate fifty-three studies that they considered landmarks in the basic science of cancer. According to their findings, published in *Nature*, they were able to reproduce the results in just six months. Earlier, Florian Prinz and his colleagues at Bayer Health Care, a German drug company, reported that they had successfully reproduced results in just a quarter of

---

[23] John Ioannidis "Why Most Published Research Findings Are False," *Public Library of Science (PLoS) Medicine* 2, no. 8 (2002).

sixty-seven seminal studies.[24] Clearly, papers with fundamental flaws live on. Despite a tenfold increase in the number of retractions over the last decade, most for use of fabricated data, they still make up no more than 0.2 percent of the 1.2 million papers published annually in scholarly journals.[25]

Medicine is overdependent on statistics. Let us consider the concept of the number needed to treat (NNT) and the pervasiveness of this concept in physician decision-making. The NNT measures the impact of a treatment by estimating the number of patients that need to be treated to have an impact on one person. David Newman, MD, provides a hypothetical situation to illustrate the concept.[26] He presents a context of heart attack victims—25 percent will die regardless of treatment, 25 percent will live regardless of treatment. The middle 50 percent is amenable to the imaginary treatment called "stop attack." When, therefore, two patients are treated with stop attack, one will survive because of the treatment. This produces an NNT of two. Before leaving what Dr. Newman calls a "straightforward" method, it would be well to point out flaws. First of all, the context is that, before administering the treatment, amenability to treatment is unknown. Further, the characteristics of the three groups are also unknown. We can assume there are differences between those who survive and those who die. What characteristic or characteristics of the "middle group" lead to amenability. We don't know. Perhaps Dr. Newman should reflect on the subtitle of his book *What Doctors Don't Know*.

In any event, the medical industry has developed numerous NNTs for specific studied interventions and drugs. According to Dr. Newman, "understanding and appreciating the NNT allows us to understand and choose the preventions and treatments, both collectively and individually, that are right for us."[27] He gives three examples of guiding care by NNTs. Mammograms, he says, have an NNT of 2,000 for preventing breast cancer death. Authorities cite far smaller NNTs. He cites the NNT for "a surgical procedure on the noncancerous breast" as five (this includes a biopsy), and the NNT for "a false positive" as

---

[24] *The Economist*, October 19, 2013, 26–28.

[25] Ibid., 28.

[26] Newman, *Hippocrates' Shadow*, 162–163.

[27] Ibid., 190.

two. Neither physician nor patient really regard a small chance of a disastrous event (death from breast cancer) as, in any way, equivalent to larger chances of far lesser outcomes. Citing the NNT for high blood pressure medicines over sixty as one hundred, he clearly discourages use of beta blockers.[28] Citing a high NNT for antibiotic treatment of strep throat in children, he discourages its use.[29]

There is a publication bias, in that there is a marked tendency of scientists and scientific journals to publish positive results and not null results. Therefore, when no effects are found, no publication occurs. This bias was first identified by the statistician, Theodore Sterling, in 1959, after he noticed that 97 percent of all published psychological studies with statistically significant data found the effect they were looking for.

---

[28] Ibid., 191.

[29] Ibid., 191.

PART V

DELIVERY OF MEDICAL CARE—CENTRAL PLANNING

Section 10

Changes in the Delivery of Medical Care

The medical industry ushered in the corporate practice of medicine

With the development of a medical industry, with corporations frequently directly controlling hospitals and clinics, providing inpatient and outpatient services, employing doctors, and setting standards and controlling costs of care, the corporate practice of medicine, long thought anathema by clinicians, became a reality.

A quintessential agency in this "corporate practice of medicine" was the Health Maintenance Organization, or HMO.

Physicians began to associate in ever larger groups for a variety of reasons.

Physicians and physician groups increasingly desired "profit centers" that could be "physician extenders" and allow escape from the billable hours problem. Whole new categories of ancillary staff were developed, including physician assistants.

A physician or a physician group could, by the simple act of employing ancillary staff, increase not only the number of procedures done, but the accompanying income. I recall an otolaryngologist on a referral panel who set up an inhalation treatment room, providing inhalation therapy for up to twenty patients with varied symptoms. The patients would be seen by the physician assistant or nurse and seated at the bench. The specialist would make rounds, "seeing" each briefly and billing for a treatment session.

Specialty groups changed the practice of medicine

Partly to compete with hospitals, specialty groups designed entirely new outpatient centers to provide a wide variety of surgical and other services. These outpatient centers do not have to achieve accreditation and do not have to adhere to such strict standards in the provision of care. The savings could be passed on to patients, but, by and large, simply augment the doctor's income.

Interventional cardiologists developed large centers devoted to angiography and the lucrative business of inserting arterial stents. Stents became so profitable that I joked with my older cardiologist who, unlike other doctors in his group, did not insert stents, that I wonder if a dog or a cat, wandering by mistake into this clinic, might not emerge with a stent or two. To my chagrin, he repeated it to the office staff as I left, blackening my reputation with the interventional cardiologists in the group.

Neurologists developed comfortable profit centers administering and interpreting electroencephalograms and myelograms.

Ophthalmologists opened "eye centers" providing cataract surgery. They developed relationships with providers of new proprietary technologies, including ever better laser machines and new replacement lenses. New proprietary lenses often had little more to offer the usually elderly patient than those paid for my Medicare, but were sold nonetheless. What elderly patient, undergoing cataract surgery, could resist "a better lens"?

Pathologists evolved into executive officers of corporations providing pathology, laboratory, and other services. Only nominally did they regard themselves as providing services to patients.

Radiologists evolved into executive officers of corporations providing imaging services. Only nominally did they regard themselves as providing services to patients.

The Technological Revolution has caused, in conjunction with our corporate structures, massive change in the delivery of health care. Just as in the Industrial Revolution, unfortunate effects and abuses had to be reined in by governmental action, so too, in the Technological Revolution, unfortunate effects and abuses will need to be reined in.

Growth of employer-based health care

By the onset of the Great Depression in the United States, there was a substantial demand for improved hospital and physician services. Charges for those services got higher and higher, increasingly out of the range of those remaining on the job in difficult times. Blue Cross developed from the employer-based health care model provided in the Baylor Plan for teachers in Texas. Periodic, relatively small payments by the employer prepaid the costs of unpredictable and expensive medical care.[30]

Growth of employer-based health care plans exploded during World War II, climbing from covering 9 percent of workers in 1940 to covering 63 percent of workers in 1953.[31] Employers, operating in the wartime context of frozen prices and wages, competed for potential employees on the basis of "benefit packages," including pensions and health care. In addition, in 1943, the Internal Revenue Service promulgated an administrative decision, later codified into law, excepting employer payments for employee health care from taxation.

Medicare

In July 1965, under the leadership of President Lyndon Johnson, Congress created Medicare to provide health care to people age sixty-five or older, without regard to medical history or income, under Title

---

[30] Melissa Thomasson, "From Sickness to Health: The Twentieth Century Development of the Demand for Health Insurance" (doctoral dissertation, 1998).

[31] Ibid.

XVIII of the Social Security Act. In 2015, Medicare was fifty years old, expanding in 1972 to cover chiropractic, physical and speech therapy. Medicare was gradually expanded to include those with disabilities receiving Social Security disability income. Under President George W. Bush, in 2003, a program covering drugs was initiated, taking effect in 2006. Medicare currently uses about thirty private insurance companies. This association formalized in 1997 under President William Clinton.

In 2010, Medicare provided coverage for 48 million people, 40 million sixty-five or over, and 8 million younger people with disabilities. This program is, in large part, paid for by a payroll tax paid equally by employers and workers.

Medicaid

Medicaid is a health care program established in 1965 under Title XIX of the Social Security Act for those with limited resources and limited income. It is jointly funded by the federal government and the states, but managed by the states. The Patient Protection and Affordable Care Act of 2010 (ACA; Obamacare) would have expanded eligibility, but the Supreme Court ruled in NFIB vs. Sibelius that this provision was coercive. Texas, Florida, Kansas, Georgia, Mississippi, and Alabama rejected participation in the expansion early, and at least seventeen other states followed.

Electronic medical records

The widespread adoption of electronic medical records that can be easily searched and compiled is another major change in the provision of medical care. Due to requirements of government and corporate payers, doctors are often to be found at a keyboard and monitor, sitting opposite the patient.

Ensuring compliance

Besides controlling the vertical system of medication production and delivery, bureaucracies are now working with the problem of ensuring compliance with "doctor's orders."[32] Only 50–70 percent of patients ever make it to a pharmacy in the first place, 40 percent fill them only once, and 50 percent discontinue after the first year. Return on investment for drugs for chronic conditions relies on improving patient compliance. The systems for improving compliance negate the physician's role and the patient's role in screening out drugs lacking efficacy or safety.

---

[32] Kalman Applebaum and Michael Oldani, eds., "Special Issue for Anthropology & Medicine: Towards an Era of Bureaucratically Controlled Medical Compliance," *Anthropology & Medicine* 17, no. 2 (2010): 113–127.

Section 11

Central Planning in Provision of Medical Care

The great political reformation, under way since at least 1980 in the United States, is being applied to health care, as to all aspects of our lives. Important tendencies and trajectories include diminishing government control which has always been, more or less, susceptible to democratic action. Instead, transfer of power and control to private entities, principally corporations, under the direct ownership and control of the rich, is under way. Those private entities seek to centralize and control all medical care. We see the elimination of horizontal or organic systems of care, substituted with systems that are hierarchical and vertical, paralleling the militarization of society. The basic themes are to impoverish everyone except the rich and further enrich the already rich.

How does a system, without empowering government control susceptible to democratic influences, manage central control? What happened is that privatized entities with an allegiance to property, not people, managed and controlled, guided by "expert systems" and "experts." Thus, horizontal networks and systems, characterizing our historical medical care, are being replaced by hierarchical vertical systems. Thus, computerized and mechanized models, lacking human concern or care, are achieving prominence. Thus, application of guidelines and algorithms creates a chimerical "objectivity" disguising decisions made by accountants on behalf of corporations and the rich.

The democratic agenda must be to retain and expand the horizontal elements of the provision of medical care, reversing the tendency to centralized ownership and control, hierarchy, and planning.

Government and insurance payment systems provided powerful new constraints on provision of medical care

With the expansion of permanent governmental and insurance company payment systems, came the development of entirely new constraints and limits on the provision of medical services.

In the United States, governmental programs, such as Medicare and Medicaid, have impinged mightily on the free market in medical care. I was a student at Indiana University Medical School when Medicare became law, and the faculty warned that such government entry into the medical field would forever change medicine.

In the United States, insurance companies experienced enormous growth after World War II.

Both governmental agencies and insurance companies determine what and who they will pay for provision of services, frequently setting up "Preferred Provider Panels," consisting of doctors who have agreed to an extensive list of constraints and limits.

Government and corporate "practice of medicine," with the assistance of "academic medicine," largely government-funded, now exerts enormous pressure on doctors to conform to centrally planned standards of care.

Head counters influence on medicine

Epidemiologists, referred to often as "head counters," sometimes in conjunction with geneticists, assumed an undue importance in the evaluation of medical care. Epidemiologists and geneticists generally work with data pools not differentiated into individual cases.

Accountants, colloquially called "bean counters," became extremely influential in the provision of health care. Choice of treatments became increasingly on the basis of cost.

Government management of expert systems

Government management of expert systems, using principles derived from the academic fields of public administration or business, has rarely been effective.

An object lesson for the United States was NASA. Early on, NASA could be thought of as a large "expert system" designed to get people into space on top of great quantities of explosives. For most of its early history, NASA was controlled, principally and directly, by astronauts and pilots.

Those experts were gradually replaced by staff with backgrounds in public administration and business. *Management*, as a discipline, depends on the premise that there is a particular expertise in managing systems, whatever those systems may be. Thus, a manager can effectively assume control of diverse systems, based upon academic training in a particular skillset. The chief executive officer of an airplane manufacturer or a computer company might, for illustration by no means rare or extreme, come from a management background at General Mills (a cereal company with no operation connected to the military or to any mill) or from a cosmetics company.

Since then, we have experienced those same bureaucrats hemming and hawing, frightened of taking action. Lacking expertise in the field, those managers are forced to rely on expensive multiply-redundant systems.

Costs have soared

Bureaucrats and managers will be allowed to "monkey around" with highly technical medical systems at our peril. A failing bureaucrat will be protected by Civil Service. A failing manager may be able to "slide laterally" to manage a fast-food company or a toy company. The medical system may even be able to rely on privacy rules to prevent public knowledge of their failure. Generally, though, repeated failures will damage the country and public trust in care.

Electronic medical records

The existence of electronic medical records allows easy surveillance of large amounts of data, being eminently searchable and compilable. They are an essential element in a centralized planning process.

Prisons and jails

With the expansion of the number in prisons and jails, the government has become the provider of all health care and all mental health care for a sizeable percentage of the population. In 2005, for example, 2,186,230 inmates were in prison or jail in the United States, of which 1,438,701 were in prison, and 747,529 were in jail. As an example of totally controlled care, the quantity and quality of medical care left a lot to be desired. Of course the criminal population was probably low on the priority list. Still, successful suits for cruel and unusual punishment, specifically, deprivation of health and mental health care, have resulted in prisons operating under court supervision in many states.

As an example, I was charged for several years to approve or disapprove prospective transfers from the California Medical Facility in Vacaville, California and the California Men's Colony in San Luis Obispo, California, to Atascadero State Hospital. There was a tendency for the prisons to want to transfer severely physically ill inmates to the mental health system, presumably to avoid paying for their medical care. I reviewed their charts. I found one inmate who had an operable brain tumor diagnosed fifteen years earlier without receiving care, then, ten years earlier, another diagnosis, but again, no care. At the time of my review, the tumor, though slow-growing, was inoperable, and was producing partial paralysis and pain. All I could do was to document the situation and send the warden a letter about it. As far as I knew, the only result was that I was relieved of my "sorting" duty.

SECTION 12

Central Regulation of Medical Care

In his farewell address on January 17, 1961, President Dwight D. Eisenhower famously warned us of a military-industrial complex. In that same address, he warned us that "public policy could itself become the captive of a scientific-technological elite."

> In the councils of government, we must guard against the acquisition of unwarranted influence, whether sought or unsought, by the military-industrial complex. The potential for the disastrous rise of misplaced power exists and will persist. We must never let the weight of this combination endanger our liberties or democratic processes. We should take nothing for granted. Only an alert and knowledgeable citizenry can compel the proper meshing of the huge industrial and military machinery of defense with our peaceful methods and goals, so that security and liberty may prosper together.
>
> . . . .
>
> Yet, in holding scientific research and discovery in respect, as we should, we must also be alert to the

equal and opposite danger that public policy could itself become the captive of a scientific-technological elite.

Arnold Relman, MD, editor of the *New England Journal of Medicine* from 1977 to 1991, commented extensively on the increasingly centralized regulation of health care till his death from melanoma in 2014. In a book entitled *Second Opinion*,[33] published in 2007, he wrote a blistering condemnation of one element of the military-industrial complex emerging after World War II, the medical industry. The medical industry is driven, he said, purely by profit motive and greed. Much that he says concerning the need to rein in the ever-increasing cost of health care in the United States is well taken. Who can deny that coverage of the presently uninsured is needed for both economic and humane reasons? Additional regulation of the insurance industry is certainly needed.

But Dr. Arnold Relman was himself a member of the scientific-technological elite about which Eisenhower cautioned us. Dr. Relman proposes to eliminate our existing health insurance system and to replace it with a governmental "single payer" system. He further proposes to replace our entire multifaceted and pluralistic system for delivery of health care with a centrally controlled, centrally planned, bureaucratic system in which physicians would be salaried workers. Who in that new system would be in charge? Most certainly government bureaucrats, advised by academic "bigwig" doctors just like Dr. Relman.

Central planning and control through "Evidence-Based Medicine"

Evidence-Based Medicine is becoming a larger and larger factor in the assessment and control of physician actions. Jerome Groopman, MD, has written extensively about this phenomenon. His latest book is *How Doctors Think*.[34]

---

[33] Arnold Relman, MD, *A Second Opinion Rescuing America's Health Care* (New York: Century Foundation Books [Public Affairs], 2007).

[34] Jerome Groopman, MD, is professor of medicine at Harvard Medical School, chief of the Division of Experimental Medicine at Beth Israel Deaconess Medical Center, and one of the world's leading researchers in cancer and AIDS. He is a staff writer for *The New Yorker* and has written for *The New York Times* and *The Washington Post*. He is author of *The*

The focus of broadcast and print media has been the alteration of the provision of health care in this country by altering the financing of health care by government and insurance companies. Neglected is the effect of those changes on the actual provision of that care.

According to Groopman, over the past decade, federal "choice architects"—i.e., doctors and other experts acting for the government and making use of comparative effectiveness—have repeatedly identified best practices. These "Best Medical Practices" are developed, choice architects tell us, through Evidence-Based Medicine, relying on Randomized Controlled Trials (RCT).

These best practices have been shown to be ineffective or even deleterious.[35] Best practices, defined by Medicare in such diverse areas as blood sugar control in hospitalized and ambulatory diabetics, congestive heart failure, kidney dialysis, hip and knee replacements, hypertension, pneumonia, and asthma caused an increased rate of death and untoward events, or, at best, had no impact.

Groopman asks, "What may account for the repeated failures of expert panels to identify and validate best practices?"[36] In my opinion, that is a question with multiple valid answers, including:

> *Measure of Our Days* (1997), *Second Opinions* (2000), *The Anatomy of Hope* (2004), and the recently released, *How Doctors Think*. Dr. Groopman holds the Dina and Raphael Recanati Chair of Medicine at the Harvard Medical School. He received his BA from Columbia College summa cum laude and his MD from Columbia College of Physicians and Surgeons in New York. He served his internship and residency in internal medicine at the Massachusetts General Hospital. Following that, his specialty fellowships in hematology and oncology were performed at the University California and the Children's Hospital/Sidney Farber Cancer Center, Harvard Medical School in Boston. Dr. Groopman served on the advisory council to the National Heart, Lung and Blood Institute for AIDS-related matters, as consultant for the Center for Biological Evaluation and Research at FDA, and a member of the Food and Drug Administration's Senior Biomedical Service Credentials Committee. He serves on many scientific editorial boards and has published more than 150 scientific articles.

[35] *New York Review of Books*, February 11, 2010, 13.

[36] Ibid. Dr. Groopman states, "Contradictory evidence reverses best practices so frequently that within one year, 15% must be changed; within

1. Excessive reliance on Evidence-Based Medicine, with the only acceptable evidence being large-scale Randomized Controlled Trials (RCT) so expensive and extensive that, by and large, only giant pharmaceutical companies are able to conduct them.
2. Excessive reliance on epidemiological data.
3. Excessive reliance on intrinsically-flawed meta-analyses.
4. Excessive reliance on statistics.

Dr. Groopman, however, points to yet another answer discussing the difference between medical practices that can be commoditized, and that can be accomplished or produced for every patient. For instance, inserting an intravenous catheter into a blood vessel is a procedure involving infection controls and using widely available equipment. If we decide to impose a "Best Medical Practice" that is an involved or complex procedure, it must be individualized. Otherwise, what we do has a great chance of lacking efficacy or safety.

An advisor to President Barack Obama, Peter Orzag, director of the Office of Management and Budget, testified as follows before the Senate Finance Committee in June 2008:

"To alter provider's behavior, it is probably necessary to combine comparative effectiveness research with aggressive promulgation of standards and changes in financial and other incentives."

According to Groopman, "The word probably is gone in the Senate health care bill. Doctors and hospitals that follow best practices as defined by government approved standards are to receive more money and favorable public assessments. Those who deviate from federal standards would suffer financial loss and would be designated as providers of poor care."[37]

It is indicative of where we are in a largely-behind-the-scenes remaking of American medicine, that the only alternative Dr. Jerome Groopman presents to authoritarian central planning is a looser central planning.

---

two years, 23% are reversed; and at 5.5 years, half are incorrect." He cites Kaveh G. Shojania, et al., in "How Quickly Do Systematic Reviews Go Out of Date: A Survival Analysis," *Annals of Internal Medicine*, August 21, 2007.

[37] Ibid., 13.

Dr. Groopman is impressed by Cass Sunstein[38] and Richard Thaler,[39] whose seminal book in the field of behavioral economics is *Nudge: Improving Decisions About Health, Wealth, and Happiness*. These experts from the University of Chicago propose "that people called 'choice architects' should redesign our social structures to protect against the incompetencies of the human mind."[40]

"The House (in contrast to the Senate bill) has explicit language repudiating such coercive measures and protecting the autonomy of the decisions of doctors and patients."[41]

Central planning and control of medical care by "guidelines" and algorithms

In the provision of medical care, treatment algorithms and treatment guidelines are becoming increasingly ubiquitous.

"Cookbook" medicine focuses on algorithms, or recipes. The patient's chief complaint becomes a proxy for the patient's entire, often

---

[38] Cass R. Sunstein (born September 21, 1954) is an American legal scholar, particularly in the fields of constitutional law, administrative law, environmental law, and behavioral economics, who currently is the Administrator of the White House Office of Information and Regulatory Affairs in the Obama administration. For twenty-seven years, Sunstein taught at the University of Chicago Law School, where he continues to teach as the Harry Kalven Visiting Professor. Sunstein is currently Felix Frankfurter Professor of Law at Harvard Law School, where he is on leave while working in the Obama administration.

[39] Richard H. Thaler (born September 12, 1945, in East Orange, New Jersey) is an American economist. He is perhaps best known as a theorist in behavioral finance, and for his collaboration with Daniel Kahneman and others in further defining that field. He currently teaches at the University of Chicago Booth School of Business and is an associate at the National Bureau of Economic Research. He has organized a series of behavioral finance seminars along with Robert Shiller, another behavioral finance expert at the Yale School of Management. Previously he taught at Cornell University and the MIT Sloan School of Management.

[40] Ibid, P. 13.

[41] Ibid, p. 13.

complicated, story, and the only focus of physician effort. The physician, thinking in a black-and-white way, wants to link that chief complaint to a clear diagnosis. A good detective does not go too quickly from the entire context of a crime. He does not concentrate only on one suspect.

Physicians quickly became aware that guidelines and "algorithms" for the provision of medical care, while ostensibly developed by academic physicians for the improvement of care, were, in reality, developed to commoditize and industrialize that care, by making the "product" manageable and uniform. Payment to the professors developing those algorithms was most often by government agencies and insurers paying for the provision of care.

Financial and other reasons, having little to do with the quality of medical care, were clearly in control.

It is easy to understand that it is folly to expect the government to manage "expert systems." It is also folly to rely on academician and statistician-developed guidelines designed to control medical practice. Central control was a proven a disaster in the USSR. We must avoid central control, whether by direct government edict or by "experts."

Central planning and control through approval to market a drug for specific indications

The Pure Food and Drug Act of 1906 was one of a series of consumer protection acts in the 20th century, establishing a federal role in food and drug packaging and purity. The law was replaced by the Federal Food, Drug, and Cosmetic Act of 1938. Increasingly, the federal administration has, in in its decisions, been influenced by pharmaceutical companies who provide information. In addition, financing of the agency is now almost entirely through payments by the companies being regulated.

In the prescribing of drugs, Food and Drug Administration (FDA) approval is more and more important.

Dr. David Graham, with the FDA for over 20 years, speaking outside his role as an associate director for science and medicine in the FDA Office of Drug Safety,[42] argued that the FDA, as currently configured, is

---

[42] "The FDA Exposed: An Interview With Dr. David Graham, the Vioxx

incapable of preventing another Vioxx or protect against unsafe drugs. It is principally interested in protecting the interests of its client, the pharmaceutical industry. The Prescription Drug Users Fee Act of 1992 sets up a system for payments to the FDA by drug companies.

The Public Citizens Health Group found that conflicts of interest were rampant in the FDA's sixteen drug committees and thirty-two other advisory panels. In 73 percent of the 221 drug reviews conducted between 2001 and 2004, there was a financial conflict of interest with the affected company or product competitors involving one or more panel members. Only 1 percent of the 3,000 panelists were recused (disqualified) within the same period, despite investments exceeding $25,000 or grants exceeding $100,000. In the case of Vioxx (and other controversial painkillers such as Celebrex and Bextra), ten members with direct links to the drug industry were on the panel that approved them.[43]

Medicines are given for "on-label indications" and "off-label indications". That is, the Food and Drug Administration (look in your encyclopedia under "Mismanaged and Unloved Minions of Big Pharma") approves medications for specific indications and those become part of the "label"—really a package insert.

So, John Q. Public and Sally S. Public read in the paper, "Two-thirds of all prescriptions are for off-label indications!" Some think, "How can doctors be so careless as to prescribe for unapproved uses?" They telephone their congresspersons and, lo and behold, a new bill pops up to prohibit prescriptions for unapproved uses. Then some medical doctor (expert) takes the congressperson into the cloakroom and whispers the facts and the bill is quietly withdrawn.

The truth is, "getting an approval for an indication" in our market system only means that some drug company has spent the millions of dollars necessary to provide the FDA with the couple of boxcars full of records of clinical trials proving the efficacy and safety of their proposed product. Now one realization that will result in a sinking feeling in

---

Whistleblower," *Life Extension*, October 2012, 67–77.

[43] Institute of Science in Society Report, January 9, 2006.

the pit of our stomachs is that the drug companies, salivating at the prospect of bonuses and profits, routinely hide outcomes unfavorable to their drugs.

But an even worse realization is that nobody takes unprofitable drugs through the approval process. Well, you ask, "Doesn't profitability mean it is a good drug, and, conversely, if a drug is not profitable, doesn't that mean it is not a good drug?" In a word repeated for emphasis—no, no, no.

Nobody takes the seven out of eight unpatentable drugs through the approval process. Nobody, for example, can patent aspirin. Nobody can patent penicillin, or tetracycline, or erythromycin, or streptomycin, etc. (on, and on, and on, and on, and on, and on).

Doctors, who have been through medical school, have more or less a handle on medicines and their indications. Remember who gets into medical school and who does not? It's not the mathematics and memory challenged who pass the MCAT and enter medical school. Those with mathematics and memory issues generally choose, you guessed it, business administration, management, and education.

So it would absolutely not be in our best interests to stop doctors from writing the two out of three prescriptions for drugs for which the indication is either off-label or there is really no label. The outcry of patients taking those drugs with efficacy and safety for decades and decades would be deafening.

Generally speaking, if we visit the local hospital emergency room or doctor's office, we can be comforted by the knowledge that things will generally go well.

What we do not realize is that things will go well, not because some important "guidelines committee," laboring away in a secret location, or because the FDA is thoroughly vetting all our medicines and medical devices. Things go well, simply put, because of doctors.

Electronic medical records

Electronic medical records allow easy surveillance of large amounts of data, being eminently searchable and compilable. They are an essential element in the centralized regulation and control of medicine. Guidelines and algorithms cease to be suggestions, and become enforceable; individual physicians can be measured for compliance with mandates for extent and type of care.

PART VI

DELIVERY OF MEDICAL CARE-FREE MARKET MECHANISMS

Section 13

The Free Market

Ronald Reagan said in his address on September 29, 1981, that: "We who live in free market societies believe that growth, prosperity and ultimately human fulfillment, are created from the bottom up, not the government down." Further, in a message to Congress on July 17, 1981, he said: "Our primary objective is simply for our citizens to have enough energy, and it is up to them to decode how much energy that is, and in what form and manner it will reach them. When the free market is permitted to work the way it should, millions of individual choices and judgments will produce the proper balance of supply and demand our economy needs."

The invisible hand is a metaphor used by Adam Smith to describe unintended benefits resulting from individual actions. The exact phrase is used just three times in Smith's writings. Market exchange automatically channeling self-interest toward socially desirable ends has been reduced in effectiveness by subsequent revolutions in industry, finance, and advertising.

Although historically and currently, the term *free market* has had and has other uses, the term means a market in which there is no intervention by the state except to enforce private ownership of property and private contracts, and no intervention by other agencies, other than the producer and the consumer. In the medical field, the consumer is best defined as a doctor-patient dyad. A free market is the opposite of a controlled market, as described in Sections 10, 11, and 12 above. In an ideal free market, property rights are voluntarily exchanged at a price arranged solely by mutual consent of sellers and buyers. By definition, buyers and sellers do not coerce each other.

We can be said to have moved into a marketing economy, where advertising has become so intense that it does not so much simply inform prospective buyers, as it coerces them into buying. A marketing economy is hostile to authentically free markets. Marketing related activities, such as advertising and branding, eat up about 50 percent of all consumer dollars, and about 1 percent of the GDP. One economist, Arthur Pigou, argued that there is too much advertising in the world, with rival companies bludgeoning each other to a standstill.

In an authentically free market, through free competition between vendors and providers of products and services, prices tend to decrease and quality of goods to increase. While a free market is not a perfect market, where individuals have perfect information, the alliance of doctors and patients in the medical field, moves it closer to that ideal.

As Milton Friedman has said, "The only way that has ever been discovered to have a lot of people cooperate together voluntarily is through the free market, and that's why it's so essential to preserving individual freedom," and, further, "The most important single central fact about a free market is that no exchange takes place unless both parties benefit."

Let us consider the market for used cars. Here, we have sellers who are individuals and buyers who are individuals. There is no intense, coercive marketing "push." Information about which cars are for sale and by whom, can come from Craigslist, or from the local equivalent of the *Pennysaver*. Both seller and buyer benefit from information available to both, as from *Consumer Reports* or from Kelly Blue Book. The buyer is able to seek a mechanic, and, essentially, form a mechanic-buyer dyad important in the final sale.

Three changes would be necessary for the medical market to be freed, as is the example above:

1. The advertising of physicians, medical devices, and drugs would need to return to being unethical.

2. Information could come from neutral sources, such as the Internet, about physician availability, medical devices, and drugs.
3. Development of doctor-patient dyads would have to be encouraged.

Transitioning to such an authentic free market would require the political will to undo or roll back the present permissive attitude toward medical advertising and to encourage the development of other neutral sources. Transitioning to an authentic free market would require the cooperation of physicians in forming doctor-patient dyads. All this will require time.

In which system would you like to live?

SECTION 14

Challenges to Free Market Mechanisms: Challenging Central Planning, Governmental or Corporate

To take back our health care, we must challenge central planning, whether governmental or corporate.

As we have seen in Part V, there have been enormous changes in the delivery of health care, in the direction of centralized planning and regulation of health care as controlled by bureaucrats, academicians, and statisticians, as well as a marked decrease in the numbers and increase in the size of providers of health care. Rolling back this "supersizing" of providers is essential to permit quality medical care at a good price. Efforts to encourage "family practice," long a policy of federal and state governments, are one approach.

The great political reformation, under way since at least 1980 in the United States, is being applied to health care, as to all aspects of our lives. We have seen the elimination of horizontal or organic systems of care with substituted systems that are hierarchical and vertical paralleling the militarization of society.

The application of guidelines and algorithms creates a chimerical "objectivity," disguising decisions made by accountants, academicians, and statisticians. Generally, "expert systems" and "experts" owe allegiance to property, not people. This allegiance has been evident in developing and using guidelines and algorithms.

With the expansion of permanent governmental and insurance company payment systems, came the development of entirely new constraints and limits on the provision of medical services.

In the United States, governmental programs, such as Medicare and Medicaid, have impinged mightily on the free market in medical care.

In the United States, insurance companies experienced enormous growth after World War II.

Both governmental agencies and insurance companies determine what and who they will pay for provision of services, frequently setting up Preferred Provider Panels consisting of doctors who have agreed to an extensive list of constraints and limits.

Government and corporate practice of medicine, with the assistance of academic medicine, largely government-funded, now exerts enormous pressure on doctors to conform to centrally planned standards of care. That pressure can be financial, with modifications of salary, payment of bonuses, or construction of a payment scale. That pressure can be through scheduling, limiting a doctor's ability to spend time with a patient.

Epidemiologists, sometimes referred to as head counters, in conjunction with geneticists, assumed an undue importance in the evaluation of medical care. Epidemiologists do not, and cannot concern themselves with individual health, but only with group or "herd" health. Their data do not lend themselves to anything else. What percentage of the total group are "outliers," not adhering to the epidemiologist's predictions? Even with the classical bell-shaped curve, that is a significant percentage.

Accountants, colloquially called bean counters, became extremely influential in the provision of health care. Accountants, controlled by such "data" as NNT (Number Needed to Treat) and NNH (Number Needed to Harm) should not be making decisions concerning provision of screening or other medical care.

Government management of expert systems, using principles derived from the academic fields of public administration or business, has rarely been effective. An object lesson for the United States was NASA. Early on, NASA could be thought of as a large expert system designed to get people into space on top of great quantities of explosives. For most of its early history, NASA was controlled, principally and directly, by astronauts and pilots. Those experts were gradually replaced by staff with backgrounds in public administration and business. Management, as a discipline, depends on the premise that there is a particular expertise in managing systems, whatever those systems may be. Thus, a manager can effectively assume control of diverse systems, based upon academic training in a particular skillset. The chief executive officer of an airplane manufacturer or a computer company might, for illustration by the extreme, come from a management background at General Mills (a cereal company with no operation connected to the military or to any mill) or from a cosmetics company. The results of this misguided system became apparent as NASA sustained failure after failure. Since then, we have experienced those same bureaucrats hemming and hawing, frightened of taking action. Lacking expertise in the field, those managers are forced to rely on multiply-redundant systems. Costs have soared.

Bureaucrats are allowed to monkey around with highly technical medical systems at our peril. A failing bureaucrat will be protected by Civil Service. A failing manager may be able to slide laterally to manage a fast-food company or a toy company. The medical system likely will hide behind patient privacy rules to prevent public knowledge of repeated failure. Generally, though, repeated failures will damage the country and public trust in care.

SECTION 15

Challenges to Free Market Mechanisms: Demographic Changes Resulting in Escalating Costs

The retirement of the baby boom generation is projected to increase Medicare enrollment from 48 million to 80 million as the number of workers per enrollee declines from 3.7 to 2.4. Medicare spending is expected to increase from 500 billion to one trillion by 2022. Medicaid provided health care to 46 million in 2001. In 2009, 62.9 million Americans were enrolled in Medicaid for at least one month. Medicaid payment assisted nearly 60 percent of all nursing home patients.

Health care spending is expected to grow at an average rate of 5.8 percent from 2012 to 2022, 1 percent faster than the growth of the GDP. Health care spending is expected to be 19.9 percent of the GDP by 2022. Medicare spending is expected to grow at an annual rate of 7.4 percent from 2015 to 2022, due to increased enrollment and utilization, increased severity of illness and treatment intensity, and faster growth in input prices partially offset by ACA mandated changes. As some states expand their Medicaid programs after 2014, an additional 8.8 million people are expected to enroll by 2016. After 2016, Medicaid spending is expected to grow by 6.6 percent a year on average, mainly driven by spending for aged and disabled beneficiaries.

These demographic and financial realities will challenge the existing free market mechanisms. Absent dramatic changes in the death rate—due perhaps to disease or war—the demographic projections are fixed. Resulting escalating costs of medical care are not fixed, but will dramatically increase, to be about one-fifth of GDP by 2022.

SECTION 16

Challenges to Free Market Mechanisms: Technology Resulting in Escalating Costs

We are in the middle of a Technology Revolution which rivals the Industrial Revolution in significance. Technological advances have dramatically changed the delivery of health care in every specialty as well as the doctor's role in that care. Physicians have become, to a greater or lesser extent, handmaidens to technology, machines, devices and drugs. Perhaps the most ubiquitous technological change was that "patent medicines" ceased to be an epithet describing elixirs, capsules, or pills sold from the back of "medicine wagons" by unscrupulous vendors. Elixirs containing "medicines," like paregoric and alcohol, had almost no efficacy for specific conditions, as well as questionable safety. Now giant pharmaceutical companies sell proprietary drugs remaining under patent for years. From patent medicine to patent medicine in a century, with the only consistency being the money to be made by the provider. The negative effects of the paregoric and alcohol in the earlier "patent medicines" were, at least, predictable. The negative effects of "modern" patent medicines are not, and often involve considerable harm.

This practice by giant pharmaceutical companies (Big Pharma) is an example of technocapitalism, discussed earlier. Professor Luis Suarez-Villa defined technocapitalism as "a new form of capitalism that is heavily grounded on corporate power and its exploitation of technological creativity. Creativity, an intangible human quality, is the most precious resource of this new incarnation of capitalism. Corporate power and profit inevitably depend on the commodification of creativity through research regimes that must generate new inventions and innovations. These regimes and the corporate apparatus in which they are embedded are to technocapitalism what the factory system and its production regimes were to industrial capitalism."[44]

Physicians and other entrepreneurs take advantage, not only of new drugs, but also of new "machines," such as the MRE, medical procedures, and medical devices. New, expensive machines require amortization, which, with often excessive self-referral of patients for testing, can occur rapidly, leaving a perpetual "profit center" for the owner.

The Technological Revolution has caused, in conjunction with our corporate structures, massive change in the delivery of health care. Just as in the Industrial Revolution, unfortunate effects and abuses had to be reined in by governmental action, so too, in the Technological Revolution, unfortunate effects and abuses will need to be reined in.

In a competitive free market system, there is a continual effort to maximize profits by lowering costs. In the medical industry, technological progress tends to increase costs.

---

[44] Luis Suarez-Villa, *Technocapitalism: A Critical Perspective on Technological Innovation and Corporatism* (Philadelphia: Temple University Press, 2009), 3.

PART VII

POSSIBLE SOLUTIONS

We must focus on the solution. If no solution is found, the tendencies and trends described above will continue. Central regulation and control of medical care will become more and more pervasive. Physicians will have less and less independence. Under the banner of "Best Medical Practice," government, corporations, and academicians will mandate their doublespeak "Best Medical Practice" without regard for what is the current and real "Best Medical Practice."

Surviving elements of the authentic free market will disappear, to be replaced by the "war of all against all" favored by the big players, in particular the insurance companies.

SECTION 17

Consumer Driven Health Care

Consumer Driven Health Care (CDHC)

Consumer-driven health care (CDHC) has been proposed as a solution to the problems discussed above. A consumer-driven health care (CDHC) system is, however, likely to founder on the complexity inherent in medicine. Physicians spend four challenging years in medical school to achieve minimal literacy in their chosen field. The "consumer" (the patient) of health care is generally not sufficiently expert to evaluate his or her needs in terms of either diagnosis or treatment. Ideally, the doctor, as an agent of the patient, and the patient, form a partnership to confront medical reality. A doctor-patient dyad is able to effectively search and find the best treatment for both chronic and acute problems.

Intrusions upon the doctor-patient relationship

The profit motive has increasingly intruded upon the doctor-patient relationship. Payments for medical care, whether by government or by insurance company, have been linked to attempts to minimize the cost of that medical care. Prior approval, involving a lengthy interaction between the doctor and the payer, is frequently required for costly diagnostic procedures, costly surgery, and costly drugs. When there is a "denial of care," it quickly becomes apparent that the playing field between doctor and payer is not level. The payer assumes the role of "decider." Historically, pressure from the medical community and from individual doctors has resulted in independent mechanisms to challenge denial of care. If there is a failure of arbitration process or medical panel to approve needed care, the ultimate challenge would involve bringing in an attorney to litigate in behalf of the doctor and the patient. Facing a potential massive judgment for wrongful death or injury, the payer is encouraged to behave in a rational and humane way.

Another intrusion upon the doctor-patient relationship has been the profit-driven effort by giant pharmaceutical companies and medical device makers to essentially "bribe" individual doctors to prescribe their expensive patented drugs or use their patented medical devices. Big drug companies have lengthy, secret lists of "consultant" doctors who receive substantial payments for little more than prescribing their drugs.

Federal legislative action is needed to eliminate egregious interference with the practice of medicine. Health care reform should include mandatory independent arbitration and review of denial of care, as well as substantial fines for insurers who delay appropriate approvals that lead to patient death or injury. Federal legislation is needed outlawing payments or benefits to doctors designed to influence medical decisions concerning care. That legislation can be modeled upon existing state legislation designed for that end.

Such regulation will outlaw behaviors in restraint of trade. Such regulation will support a continued competitive market evaluation of diagnostic and treatment efforts by the best "medical team"—the doctor-patient team. Such regulation will permit doctors to continue in their role as expert ombudspersons, speaking and acting on behalf of their patients.

Existing regulations limiting corporate practice of medicine must be strengthened. This country has had enough of profit-driven corporations and agencies wreaking havoc in financial services. Now they have been unleashed to wreak havoc in medicine. Only individual licensed physician should be able to perform surgery and prescribe drugs.

The health care industry has long resented the independent role of physicians. Physicians have had to fight protracted and intense battles, particularly in settings where they are salaried, to maintain their independence. It would be disingenuous not to accede that independence has the effect of increasing remuneration to doctors. It would, however, be wrong to believe physician independence is not also cherished for its role in permitting physicians to continue to act on behalf of those coming to them for care.

Insuring quality of care

What many do not realize is that things go fairly well now, and will continue to go fairly well in the foreseeable future, not because some important "guidelines committee," staffed by bureaucrats and academics, is laboring away in some secret location, or because the Food and Drug Administration is thoroughly vetting all our medications and our medical devices, but because individual doctors have consciences and ethics. Quality of care will ultimately be dependent on the free market evaluation of treatments by relatively independent doctor-patient teams.

Historically and globally, we have had huge and tragic experiments with central governmental planning and control. On such failed experiment was the USSR. Khrushchev is said to have cried entering supermarkets in the United States during a visit. The Soviet Union fell by its own weight.

Which system produces the best medical care?

Individual doctors

But individual doctors have been soldiering on, struggling and working with their patients to improve the quality of their lives and extend their lives.

Despite the corporate flacking and flogging of expensive proprietary techniques, devices, and drugs, doctors and patients continue, in the real world, to evaluate what works and what helps. This is the real competitive marketplace—far from corporate-funded research, far from corporate-funded guidelines and algorithms, and far from corporate-paid advertising of the latest expensive device or drug.

This competitive marketplace is still robust. It is still alive and well.

SECTION 18

DELIVERY OF MEDICAL CARE- PHYSICIAN'S ROLE

Challenges to the Independence of Physicians

Physicians have experienced numerous challenges in the changing environment for the delivery of health care.

Reformation of medical education

Following the release of the "Flexner Report," a study by Abraham Flexner, in 1910, there was a major reform in medical education. Recently, medical schools have continued to change, steadily, though slowly influenced by entrepreneurial and technological concerns. Unsurprisingly, these changes have moved in the direction of empowering academicians and medical schools, at the expense of clinicians. Advancement and tenure for faculty became principally dependent on the acquisition of research grants.

Doctors less homogeneous and more diverse

The United States has become less homogeneous and more diverse during the last century. As a group, doctors are also less homogeneous and more diverse. Medicine is no longer the province of the white male born in this country. International medical graduates (IMGs) constitute about 25 percent of all doctors. Just under 20 percent of IMGs are from India. Eleven other countries contribute from 2 percent to 9 percent of the total: Philippines, Mexico, Pakistan, Dominican Republic, Russia, Grenada, Egypt, Korea, Italy, China, and Iran. Foreign medical graduates are more and more influential. Minorities speak with a louder voice.

Physicians as salaried employees

University medical centers provide a wide range of services and employ doctors who are frequently on the medical school teaching staff.

Health Maintenance Organizations (HMOs) emerged as an alternative model for delivery of health care.

Corporations provide an increasing proportion of our health care.

Hospitalists, and salaried employees of hospitals, have emerged as a separate specialty.

Physicians as entrepreneurs

Physicians have been encouraged to view themselves as businessmen attempting to maximize their income. This has not been a negative development to the extent that it has meant increasing the quantity of services or the quality of care.

Too frequently, however, reimbursement schedules, whether by government or insurance company payers, have come to exercise an undue influence on treatment choices.

Physician specialists have developed practices depending on particularly well reimbursed procedures

Psychopharmacology and psychotherapy—"pills" or "talk" are two modes of intervention in psychiatry. Prescription of psychotropic medications is very well reimbursed, requiring less physician time. Psychotherapy not only is, on an hourly basis, far less well reimbursed, but also requires repeated "justifications" eating up non-reimbursed physician time.

Electroconvulsive therapy (ECT) had, until recently, been particularly well reimbursed. When I began work at Edgemont Hospital in Hollywood, California, over 85 percent of all patients received ECT. ECT, like surgery, was a discrete operation—requiring anesthesia—with moderately well-studied short-term effects. Newly out of my residency, I was from the *One Flew Over the Cuckoo's Nest*[45] generation, and quickly changed that.

Injudicious application of cost control mechanisms by government or insurance company payers can negatively impact quality of care

Physicians have been rewarded for selecting inexpensive treatments and punished for selecting costly ones.

Primary care

Reliance on physician specialists and technology has minimized the role of the primary care physician.

---

[45] Ken Kesey, *One Flew Over the Cuckoo's Nest* (New York: Signet Books, 1962).

SECTION 19

Choice for Physicians: Aesculapius or Mercury

Physicians must choose either a professional or a market model of practice. On December 9, 2009, Andrew Weil, MD, at the Anaheim Convention Center, gave a keynote address to over 7,000 attendees, mostly doctors, psychologists, and therapists, from all over the world— from the United States, Europe, South America, Africa, Russia, India, China, Japan, and Australia. His topic was "Integrative Medicine: The Mind-body Connection and the Future of Health Care." Dr. Weil was careful to point out that integrative medicine was not "complementary" or "alternative" medicine, but attempted to integrate traditional Western medicine with other perspectives and approaches. Dr. Weil has been on the cover of *Time Magazine* twice, and he is an impressive speaker. One of his early points was that legislation that has currently passed both Senate and House is about insurance company reform and not about health care. He believes health care is in a crisis. He believes that:

- The focus should not be on treating disorders but on healing.
- The focus should be on the mind-body.
- The doctor-patient relationship should be at the heart of medicine.
- Excessive reliance on technology should be eschewed.
- Other culture's mostly low-technology healing systems and methods should be explored.

Evidence-Based Medicine, while the phrase initially sounds good, as presently discussed, relies almost exclusively on randomized controlled studies, which (1) are prohibitively expensive and thus mostly financed by giant pharmacology companies, and 2) are simplified to a single variable and thus divorced from practice of medicine in the real world. Evidence-Based Medicine neglects other evidence. Dr. Weil said that Evidence-Based Medicine might be described by some as a "conspiracy" by pharmacology companies. He said that Evidence-Based Medicine is "a new fundamentalism."

Dr. Weil sees conventional medicine as driven by technology and the profit motive, both having unfortunate consequences as well as benefits. The profit motive destroys the doctor-patient relationship.

Dr. Weil decried the current identification of *medicine* with *drugs.* He referred briefly to the derivation of the word *medicine.* Medicine comes to English from the Latin, *medicina,* and refers to the art practiced by the *medicus* or physician. The Latin word itself may well derive originally from the root, media, referring to a middle way, or balance, since in classical Greek medicine (that which was known and practiced in the Roman world), health was a matter of balance, and disease was understood as an imbalance of the body (or of the bodily fluids, called "humours"). This balance could be restored by a medicus.[46]

---

[46] The website, PandoraWordBox.com, has an interesting reflection on the word, *medicine*. [This material was not part of Andrew Weil's keynote address, but is interesting in its own right.]
Thus far in the Western world, Aesculapius, or Esculapius, continues to be the central representation of the Arts and Sciences of Medicine....
... The staff or the caduceus of Esculapius has only one intertwined snake, in contrast to the caduceus of mercenary Mercury sporting two vipers. Perhaps the sole reptile on the staff of Esculapius denotes that the physician has the fiduciary duty to only serve the interests of his patient, a fundamental tenet of medical ethics. Perhaps physicians who view their patients as "clients" should also alter their caduceus by adding an extra viper which is consonant with the emblem of "caviat emptor" implying two parties without trust for each other.

SECTION 20

Patients and Doctors

Traditionally, medicine had been a profession or guild, providing services in a market environment. Provision of services was primarily on the basis of free market principles. Price generally varied depending on the elements of supply and demand. Medical care began with a patient's verbal history and an examination of the body part. The individual physician then did everything possible to provide rapid relief.

A decentralized, robust system of competition has somehow managed to survive through the practice choices of individual doctors, in conjunction with their patients.

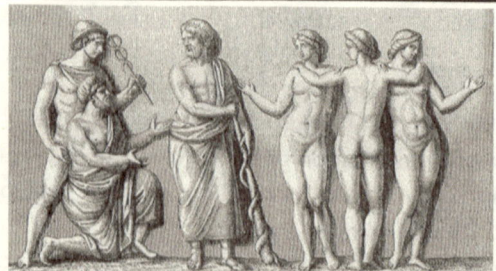

Esculapius (Representing Medicine) between Mercury (Merchants) and the Graces (Medicine, Hygiene and Panacea) [Esculapius treated Patients while Merchants make deals with Clients]

A patient-doctor dyad is required to insure the best available care for the individual patient. The patient lacks the expertise required to survey available treatments and to choose the best for him or her (see Part VI, Consumer Driven Health Care). The doctor and the patient need transparency to allow the doctor to account for the patient's wishes and to allow the patient to access the doctor's expert guidance. Together, the patient-doctor dyad can challenge the hierarchical structures, and, with thousands of such dyads, permit a true free market to exist, organized on a horizontal region-wide basis.

The emergence of the Internet, and the ready availability of information concerning specific disorders, has already affected the patient-doctor dyad, as has advertising of treatments, particularly drugs. Patients and doctors can discuss what is best for the patient, from this sea of treatments, avoiding the unadvertised and advertised sharks in that sea.

Each doctor, in conjunction with colleagues, sharing experiences in their individual practices will bring to the discussion far more than is available in "continuing medical education" courses traditionally weighted by the financing by "providers."

Informed consent will, thus, become far more genuinely informed than is presently true.

Section 21

Physician Negotiation with Payers

The physician, acting as an agent of the patient, can negotiate with payers, whether governmental or corporate. Lucien Roberts, III, MHA, FACMPE, executive director of Neuropsychological Services of Virginia, and a consultant to medical groups, has developed a "report card" for payers. He describes the process as follows:[47]

> There are many intangibles to consider before sitting at the table with a payer to negotiate reimbursement. Effectively evaluated and presented, these intangibles can bring a tangible value to your payer negotiations. Further, if you involve your staff in a discussion of these intangibles, not only will you get their buy-in, but you will learn things that may help you during negotiation. My practice uses an informal payer report card that has become a key source of intangible information that we use to good effect when negotiating with payers. Next to my miter saw and my cordless drill, the payer report card is my favorite tool, and it has been invaluable in

---

[47] Lucien Roberts, III, MHA, FACMPE, is executive director of Neuropsychological Services of Virginia. He also consults with medical groups and doctors in areas such as compliance, physician compensation, negotiation, strategic planning, billing, and collections. He may be reached at lucien.roberts@yahoo.com.

payer negotiations. Simply put, the payer report card is a template that is used to rank each of my payers on an "A" to "F" basis; there is a comment field next to each payer's grade where comments on what is liked/disliked about the payer can be added. I ask each employee—front office, clinical staff, business office, physicians—to rank the payers from his or her perspective. The results are subjective, but irrefutable—your team is letting you know which payers make it easiest, or hardest, to provide good patient care.

. . . .

Knowledge is power. Knowing the good, the bad, and the ugly about your practice's relationship with its payers strengthens your hand and can give you a new edge at the negotiating table.

Negotiations are impossible if the "power gradient" is too great. Corporations did not negotiate with employees until they unionized, reducing the ability of the corporations to run roughshod over workers. Doctors, unable now to negotiate due to refusal of government or corporate payers to negotiate, will need to form regional groups speaking with a single voice.

Independent practice associations (IPAs) have been around since the 1950s, negotiating to provide services at a competitive rate, providing benefits for physicians and patients alike. Since 2001, however, the Federal Trade Commission (FTC) and the Department of Justice (DOJ) have prosecuted thirty-six IPAs, representing 18,000 physicians, for the "crime" of price-fixing, or negotiating with payers. The success of these prosecutions has hinged on the enormous cost to an IPA to engage the FTC and DOJ in court. The FTC and the DOJ have practically unlimited legal resources, the IPAs, relatively—far, far less.

Academicians' control professional organizations, and have a vested interest in denying clinicians power in the system. Academicians retain the most power when the clinician must march to the tune of the government and corporate payers and comply with their "guidelines" and mandates.

Central Planning and Control vs. Free Market Mechanisms in Medicine, Leo Ingle, M.D., October 10, 2009

My personal experience with negotiating with insurers came in Fairbanks, Alaska. The context was one of a shortage of physicians, particularly specialists. Insurance companies varied in their requirements, some requiring authorization in advance, some requiring regular justifications for continued treatment. One particular insurance company was particularly uncooperative. My filings for reconsideration were ignored. Finally, I decided to take no new patients for whom payment would be by that insurer. A particular patient was referred to me by them four times—each time, I said no, politely. I was called several times and finally said I chose not to deal with them. I learned that I was the only specialist in the entirety of Northern Alaska available to them. They would, if I persisted in refusing to treat their patients, have to fly them to Anchorage for care, entailing a great deal of expense. Before taking that patient, and those that followed, I demanded and received an apology and payment for all the cases they had denied. Going forward, they made reasonable adjustments, and became a good "customer." Insurance companies will respond to a reality "on the ground." Rarely does a physician have the leverage I possessed, however.

PART VIII

DISTRIBUTED MEDICAL EDUCATION

Section 22

Distributed Medical Education

The Flexner Report is a book-length study of medical education in the United States and Canada, written by Abraham Flexner and published in 1910 under the aegis of the Carnegie Foundation. Flexner visited 155 medical schools from December 1908 to April 1910. He developed a conceptual model of how medical education should be conducted. Publication of the report resulted in denial of recognition by licensing boards of poor schools, and the reduction of the total number of medical schools from 133 in 1910 to 85 ten years later.

Such an effort to set standards differs from the central control of medical education by government and corporations. Just as government and corporations sought to control the "medical industry," they also realized a need to control the educations of individual workers in that "industry." Faculty at each school achieved recognition and tenure by participating in government and corporate financing of research projects. Academicians were being prepared to participate in the control of clinical work.

The challenge for medical colleges, which share in the same processes as medicine in general, is to deal with the demand for well-educated graduate doctors. According to the American Medical Association's masterfile for 2010, there are currently about 240,000 primary care physicians in the United States. Adjusting to include those professionally active and exclude the retired, there are 233,403 doctors. Of these, 25 percent are international medical graduates (IMGs). The increase in the percentage of IMGs was largely due to immigration changes in the 1990s.

According to the American Association of Medical Colleges, there will be a shortage of 130,600 physicians by 2025, of which 65,800 will be primary care physicians.

There is certainly a need for a new Flexner Report and rapid enactment of its recommendations. Medical education, though adhering to professional standards, must be independent of governmental and corporate control. Financing must be made available from sources imposing no constraint on research findings. Such financing must maintain adequate incomes for faculty and permit reasonable tuition and fees for students. Government financing, based on the number of either entering or graduating medical students, would meet that need, as far as faculty salaries are concerned.

Tuition and fees for attending medical school have gone up. According to the American Association of Medical Colleges, for the 140 accredited United States Medical Schools reporting for the academic year 2014–2015, tuition and fees were $28,719 a year, or $114,876 for four years at public schools for residents, and $49,000 a year or $196,000 for four years. Tuition and fees for private schools were $47,673 a year or $190,692 for four years. This burden, resulting in enormous student debt, coupled with the low pay during internship and residency, virtually eliminates doctor choice. The doctor must become an entrepreneur in order to pay down debt. Government financing is needed. I attended Indiana University Medical School, entering in 1963 and graduating in 1967. Thanks to funding of Indiana University Medical School by the State of Indiana, my tuition was only $200 a semester, or $400 a year, throughout the entire four years. Had my tuition been much more, I would not have been able to attend.

Traditional instructor-centered teaching is yielding more and more to a learning-centered model that puts learners in control of their own learning. E-learning refers to the use of Internet technologies to deliver a broad array of solutions that enhance knowledge and performance. Its use has gained popularity in the past decade, but its use is highly variable among medical schools. Students see e-learning as complementing traditional instructor-led methods, such as lectures, forming part of a blended-learning strategy.

Expansion of existing medical schools, independent of central control and adopting a blended-learning strategy, appears to offer one solution to the requirement for more physicians.

Such an educational system would be more likely, in the large group of independent schools, to discover and test alternative treatments proven valuable in recent years.

PART IX

ALTERNATIVE TREATMENTS

SECTION 23

Alternative Treatments

Alternative treatments arise and flourish in a system with relaxed central regulations and controls. In a genuine free market system, each alternative treatment stands or falls on its own merits, and not on its capacity to make money for providers. In a genuine free market system, each physician-patient dyad, choosing from the universe of possible treatments, will choose the one or more best suited to the individual person.

Alternative treatments include:

Indian medicine

The origins of the Ayurveda, evolving from the Vedas, have been traced back to 5,000 BC, originating as oral teachings and later as medical texts. Ayurvedic medicine is a system of Hindu traditional medicine. By the medieval period, Ayurvedic practitioners had developed a number of medicinal preparations and surgical procedures for the treatment of various disorders. Ayurveda enumerates seven basic tissues: plasma, blood, muscles, fat, bone, marrow, and semen. Ensuring the proper function of channels that transport bodily fluids leads to treatment with massages using oils. Ayurveda deals with plant-based medicines and treatment. A variety of alcoholic beverages is used in Ayurveda, as well as purified opium from the poppy. Apart from the Ayurveda, Yoga, as practiced in India, is another system of Hindu traditional medicine.

In Santayana/Hindu, tantric, and yogic traditions, *chakras* are energy nodes in the subtle body. W. Brugh Joy, MD, a specialist in internal medicine, developed a system of treatment through "manipulation" of those chakras.[48]

Chinese medicine

Traditional Chinese medicine is based upon traditions of more than 2,000 years, including various forms of herbal medicine, acupuncture, massage, exercise, and dietary therapy. Traditional Chinese medicine postulates that the body's vital energy or chi, circulates through channels, called meridians, to functional entities that regulate digestion, breathing, aging, etc. It is primarily used as a complementary or alternative treatment approach. *Chinese Natural Cures: Traditional Methods for Remedies and Prevention*, by Henry C. Lu, is a beautifully silk-bound example of the bookmaker's art, describing traditional Chinese medicine.[49]

Anthroposophical medicine

In 1921, Austrian philosopher, Rudolf Steiner, applied anthroposophical principles to the field of medicine. In 1925, with Dr. Ita Wegman, he published *Fundamentals of Therapy: An Extension of the Art of Healing Through Spiritual Knowledge*. According to Dr. Richard Fried, president of the Physicians Association for Anthroposophic Medicine, "We are trying to add a wider image of the interplay of physical and spiritual factors in illness and health, in addition to the effects of environment, heredity, individual destiny and karma." Included among anthroposophical therapies are healing mineral baths, air, light, and warmth treatments, rhythmic massage, and the dance-like eurhythmy.

---

[48] William Brugh Joy, *Joy's Way: A Map for the Transformational Journey: an Introduction to the Potentials for Healing with Body Energies* (J.P. Tarcher, 1979).

[49] Henry C. Lu, *Chinese Natural Cures: Traditional Methods for Remedies and Prevention* (New York: Black Dog & Leventhal, 1986).

Homeopathic medicine

Homeopathic medicine is a system of alternative medicine created in 1796, based upon the doctrine of "like cures like," whereby a substance that causes symptoms and signs of disease in normal people will cure similar symptoms and signs in sick people. Associated with this, is the practice of using very small doses of selected drugs.

Chiropractic

Chiropractic, the largest alternative medicine profession, is a system based upon manipulation of the musculoskeletal system. Chiropractic is well-established in the United States and Canada, overlapping with osteopathy, massage, and physical therapy. D.D. Palmer founded chiropractic in the 1890s. Following a successful antitrust suit in 1987, third party payers are prohibited from discriminating against chiropractic.

Supplements

Supplements have emerged as a major alternative treatment to prevent illness and promote health. Substances, called "nutriceuticals," are taken regularly, for a wide variety of reported ills. While I take over fifty supplementary softgels, capsules, or tablets a day, I believe that the following ten supplements (twenty softgels, capsules, or tablets) are best supported by available evidence:

TEN "EVIDENCE BASED" SUPPLEMENTS

SUPPLEMENT	BRAND AND FORM	DAILY DOSE
OMEGA-3 FATTY ACIDS	Nature's Bounty Fish Oil, containing 980 mg of Omega 3 in 1400 mg. Omega-3 in form of DHA, 650 mg and EPA, 250 mg	Four softgels a day, for 2.6 g of DHA and 1.0 g of EPA
CoQ-10*	Kirkland CoQ-10, 300 mg and Quinol (Ubiquinol), 100 mg (a more active form of CoQ-10)	One softgel of each a day

Resveratrol	Swanson's Vitamins, Resveratrol, 500 mg (the active ingredient in red grapes and red wine)	One capsule a day
Vitamin C	Kirkland Vitamin C, 1000 mg, with Rose Hips and Citrus Bioflavinoid Complex	One or two tablets a day
Vitamin D**	Nature's Bounty, D-3, 5000 IU	One to three softgels a day
Vitamin E***	Swanson's Vitamins, Full Spectrum E with Tocotrienols	One softgel a day
Vitamin K	Life Extension, Super K with Advanced K-2 Complex Containing 1000 mcg of K-1 and 1200 of K-2 (Although expensive, Life Extension is the only supplier of this high dose of Vitamin K.)	Three tablets a day
Vitamin B-12	Nature Made, B-12, 1,000 mg	One tablet a day
Calcium, Magnesium and Zinc	Country Life Cal-Mag-Zinc, containing, in three tablets, calcium, 1000 mg, magnesium, 500 mg, and zinc, 50 mg	Three tablets a day
Folate	Swanson's Vitamins, Folate, 5-methyltetrahydrofolic acid, 800 mcg	One capsule a day

*While not in "top ten," CoQ-10 is more effective when combined with Acetyl L-Carnitine, 500-1000 mg a day.

**I monitor the blood level of Vitamin D, and target a level of 50 to 80.

***Avoid vitamin E products containing only alpha tocopherol. That ingredient (far cheaper to manufacture and buy) may actually be harmful in higher doses, while the recommended product is high in gamma tocopherol and has the full range of tocopherols and tocotrienols.

Medical schools and physicians are overwhelmingly hostile to nutritional medicine.

Food Safety

In Chinese medicine above, the efficacy for attaining good health by balancing the properties of foods was mentioned. *Chinese Natural Cures* details that process.[50] In supplements above, the efficacy for attaining good health by taking appropriate supplements was discussed. Modifying diet to deal with food sensitivities and allergies is emerging as another alternative treatment, one focusing, not on the efficacy of foods for health, but on the safety of diet. A core concept is the "allergen burden," consisting of all the allergens to which the lungs, the gut, and the skin are exposed. Individuals vary in the burden or load of allergens the body can tolerate before symptoms and signs are experienced—often asthma or a rash. A "reactor" is sometimes said to be atopic.

In 1968, at Mobile General Hospital, I admitted a young nine-year-old boy with a history of intractable asthma. He had had nineteen previous hospital admissions with difficult-to-treat asthma. After his acute symptoms were resolved, I elected, after discussion with the concerned parents, to undertake a food elimination diet. Such a diet is difficult, since the foods to be eliminated are ubiquitous. First, we eliminated dairy products, with neither improvement in his asthma nor response to a challenge meal. Then we eliminated wheat and wheat products. After eliminating those foods, he had a robust response to a challenge meal. With a dietary change, elimination of wheat and wheat products, he remained symptom-free for the duration of follow-up.

Food elimination diets are not usual, except in a life-threatening situation. The ability to test for allergies was needed. Until recently, testing has not been very helpful. Skin prick tests were all that was available for many years, and only revealed IgE mediated responses. Principal antibodies measured are IgE (immunoglobulin E) and IgG (immunoglobulin G). Of particular concern is the IgG, not the rapid-acting IgE, responsible for acute allergic reactions.

---

[50] Ibid.

The radioallergosorbent (RAST) test and the enzyme-controlled immunoassay test were a great improvement. The Food Safe Allergy Test, available from Meridian Valley Lab, uses the enzyme-linked immunosorbent assay (ELISA), developed in 1976.

Dance therapy

Dance has traditionally been thought to have healing properties. While at Edgemont Hospital in Hollywood in the 1970s, I organized a program of movement and dance therapy in conjunction with the occupational therapist. I was impressed with it, believing it to "free" participants to benefit from other modalities.

Music therapy

Sound has traditionally been thought to have healing properties. Brugh Joy, MD, held therapy groups in his Feather Mountain Conference Center, in Prescott, Arizona, relying on intense sound.[51] Groups of perhaps two dozen men and women would sit on mats in an otherwise empty room. Four giant speakers in the corners of the room would play meditational music at levels approaching pain. Participants reported both hallucinatory experiences as well as healing.

---

[51] Ibid.

PART X

COST CONTAINMENT

Section 24

Cost Containment

Restoring the free market in medicine

An otherwise excellent book on medical care in the United States, *Hippocrates' Shadow*,[52] by David H. Newman, MD, falls prey to a common myth about medicine. He says, "In the United States we have chosen a health care system controlled by the invisible hand of market forces."[53] Section 2, above, describes non-market constraints and limits on provision of medical services, including the appearance and actuality of the utility of those services, humanitarian concerns, and medical ethics. Section 5, above, differentiates a competitive free market system where there is a continual effort on the part of competitors to improve the technical forces of production in order to maximize profits by lowering costs with the medical industry where commodities are not standardized, and where technological progress tends to increase costs, rather than lower costs. Sections 11 and 12, above, describe central planning in medical care and central regulation of it. Sections 13, 14, 15, and 16 describe the free market and the enormous challenges to free market mechanisms. Sections 18, 19, and 20 discuss the physician's role in the changing field. Many fall prey to confusion about the current system. The term *"Free Market"* has been subjected to doublespeak though the current system is neither a "market" nor "free." Restoring

---

[52] *Op. cit.*

[53] Ibid., 196.

a genuine market in medical care, in which consumers choose from an array of products, varying in nature, quality, and price, is the subject of this book.

Technocapitalism

Technocapitalism, defined elsewhere, drives up medical costs in two ways: first, an excessive number of drugs, procedures, and tests are prescribed, and, secondly, the costs of those drugs, because of national, regional, or local, monopolies, are excessive.

Reliance on Randomized Controlled Trials

Reliance on Randomized Controlled Trials, developed in 1948, has provided an expensive way to guide medical care. Less expensive observational trials, observation, and anecdote have been virtually replaced. Compare, for example, the cost of Plavix and the cost of aspirin, both drug thinners. Plavix costs $3.22 a pill, whereas aspirin four cents a pill. Further, long-term use of Plavix has not been tested, but aspirin has been prescribed for centuries.[54] Ironically, 30 percent of the population is non-responsive to Plavix, making it costly not only in terms of dollar cost, but in terms of unexpected and potentially catastrophic failure.

Similar procedures and care have widely varying costs

Medical bills for the same procedure vary widely. A study published in the *Annals of Internal Medicine* reported on the results of analysis of data submitted to the state on 19,368 patients with appendicitis. Only patients eighteen to fifty-nine years old, having uncomplicated cases with hospital stays of less than four days, were considered. Bills varied from $1,529 to $182,955—with many well over $100,000 and under $2,000.

---

[54] Stephanie Nano, "Compared to Aspirin, Plavix Not Worth the Cost," *Los Angeles Times*, June 10, 2002.

Containment is essential

The United States currently spends 16 percent of its GDP on health care, and is theoretically on track to spend 100 percent of its GDP by 2065.

We cannot continue to expend ever-increasing amounts on medical care. The central regulation and control of medicine by government and insurers has been a major element in that runaway spending. The interference with the mechanisms of the free market has been another. Modifying the role of the physician to that of an entrepreneur rather than an agent of the patient has been another.

PART XI

SECTION 25

Conclusions

It's time to "take back our health care," restoring the traditional free market in medical care. As with any revolution, the revolution in medicine that would take back our health care would be meaningless if there were no replacement planned. This book, taken in its entirety, described a replacement system relaying on an authentic free market.

The term *doublespeak* has its origin in George Orwell's book, *Nineteen Eighty-Four*. Although the term doublespeak is not used in Orwell's book, it is a close relative of one of the book's central concepts, "doublethink." Orwell highlights examples: peace is war, freedom is slavery, and love is hate. In medicine, examples are the capture of phrases, which are then redefined to mean exactly what the system wants them to mean. For example, "Best Medical Practice" is redefined to mean what government, corporations, and academicians want it to mean—a static, measurable, "expert-generated," government-and-insurer-approved entity, instead of the fluid concept traditionally part of the medical lexicon. Section 8 describes the pirating of previously conceived "Best Medical Practice." Similarly, free market is no longer the concept described by Adam Smith in *Wealth of Nations*, but a never ending war of all-against-all, where "the advantage" is not the mutually beneficial and benign "comparative advantage" of Smith, but gleanings of greed, snatched by victors in the struggle.

The House of Medicine is built on the shifting sand of "Best Medical Practice" and research. The "Best Medical Practice" in the governmental, corporate, and academic meaning changes with too great a rapidity to be of much utility. Best Medical Practice," as determined by the free market (and not by government, by corporations, or by academicians), is sufficiently fluid to keep up with changing science and technology.

As discussed in Section 9, the results of Randomized Controlled Trials (RCTs), cannot replace observational studies, observation, or anecdote. The judgment of clinicians is a far better guide. Medical practice must rely on a variety of inputs.

There are several themes running through this book. The most prominent theme is the restoration of a genuine free market in medical care—not the market touted by corporations, but a market more akin to the traditional free market and Greek and medieval medical care. Even free markets operate under constraints, the fewer the better— these have traditionally included science, humanitarian, and ethical concerns.

The context today includes the amazing scientific and technological advances in medicine, as well as the systems for their development and deployment. Medicine, in utilizing technology, needs to consider people as well as profit. In Part II, Section 5, we explored scientific and technological advances in medical care. We described the history of these advances in the field of medical care. We introduced the concept and term, technocapitalism. We described multiple effects of these scientific and technological advances in changing the role of physicians and in increasing costs of care. Areas of technology, to include medical devices, vaccines, and drugs were discussed. The effects of computers and electronic medical records on medical care were discussed.

In Part II, Section 6, we discussed the development and deployment of technological advances, especially the long delay in the spread across the nation.

In Part II, Section 7, we described how the dichotomy of patients and profits operated to the benefit of neither.

Changes in the delivery of medical care have resulted in increasingly centralized control and regulation of medical care. These changes are considered in Section 10, Section 11, and Section 12. In Part V, Section 10, we described the changes in the delivery of medical care. In Part

V, Section 11, we described the emerging centralized planning process in the delivery of medical care. In Part V, Section 12, we described the emerging regulation of medical care and its delivery.

Changes in the delivery of medical care have provided challenges to free market mechanisms. In Part VI, we described the free market and challenges to it:

In Section 13, we described the free market.

In Section 14, we discussed dealing with central planning, governmental or corporate.

In Section 15, we discussed the effect of demographic changes on medical costs.

In Section 16, we discussed the effect of technological changes on medical costs.

Changes in the delivery of medical care have resulted in challenges to the independence of doctors. In Part VII, Section 18, we discussed the role of independent physicians in providing a solution.

Doctors are presented with a choice of serving people or seeking profit. In Part VII, Section 19, "Aesculapius or Mercury," we presented the choice confronting physicians: either focus primarily on their practice as a business, making profits, or focus primarily on excellence of patient care. A practicing doctor gets to choose how long he or she will spend with each patient, potentially doubling income by cutting face-to-face time in half. A practicing doctor can make more money by avoiding difficult cases and scheduling easy cases. A practicing doctor can maximize income by avoiding unreimbursed services, such as family interviews and telephone calls. A practicing doctor can maximize income by avoiding time-consuming emergency care. Increasingly, a patient with an emergency calls his doctor, to hear, "If you have an emergency, call nine-one-one." Not so many years ago, this would have been thought of as abandoning the patient. Unfortunately, as discussed in Section 22, on medical education, presently, doctors, facing enormous student debt, have little real choice.

The dyad of the physician and the patient, exercising free choice in a wide universe of options, represents the best chance for restoring the free market in medical care existing before 1600. In Part VII, Section 20, we described the physician-patient dyad, the core concept in the proposed solution.

In Part VII, Section 17, we discussed difficulties with an occasionally proposed solution to the problems discussed above, "Consumer Driven Health Care."

Physicians and physician groups must be free to negotiate payment from government and corporate payers. In Part VII, Section 21, we discussed the role of the physician as an agent for the patient in negotiating with insurers.

Cost containment will be real only in the context of this restored free market in medical care (Section 24).

We must focus on the solution. If no solution is found, the tendencies and trends described above will continue. Central regulation and control of medical care will become more and more pervasive. Physicians will have less and less independence. Under the banner of "Best Medical Practice," government, corporations, and academicians will mandate their doublespeak "Best Medical Practice" without regard for what is the current and real "Best Medical Practice."

Surviving elements of the authentic free market will disappear, to be replaced by the "war of all against all" favored by the big shark-like players, especially the insurance companies.

It is time to *take back our health care,* restoring the free market in medical care.

www.ingramcontent.com/pod-product-compliance
Lightning Source LLC
Chambersburg PA
CBHW030816180526
45163CB00003B/1309